AROMATHERAPY RECIPES
using Pure Essential oils
Volume 1

By
Penny Keay
2008

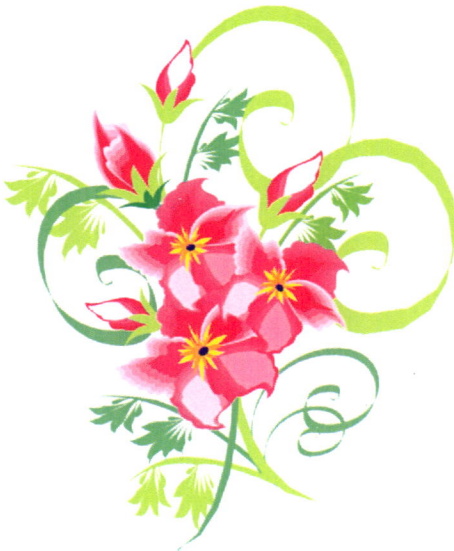

First Printing—November 2008 (100)

First Published in the United States in 2008
By Penny Keay
2898 County Road 103
Barnum, MN 55707-8808

Graphics and Clip art courtesy and with permission (Royalty Free) from Clipart.com by Jupeter Images.

ISBN 978-0-9822142-0-6
Printed in the U.S.A.

Acknowledgement and Thanks

A Thank you to everyone interested in Aromatherapy. As I helped you, many of these recipes were a result of helping those that asked for recipes and blends for specific health concerns.

A Special Thank you to my husband, Alan, for sparking an interest in Aromatherapy and the study of essential oils in both of us.

An Extra Special Thank you to Jaylene, who without the many hours of typing, design and layout this book would not have been possible.

Thank you Everyone,

Penny

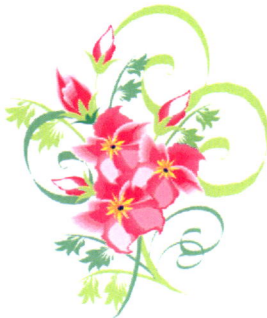

AROMATHERAPY RECIPES
using Pure Essential oils
Volume 1
By Penny Keay

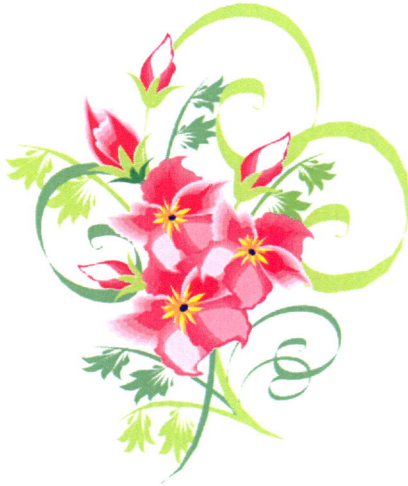

DISCLAIMER:

The information and recipes in this book when used in conjunction with a known health concern are not to be used without the diagnosis and knowledge of your Health Care Practioner.

All recommendations, suggestions and recipes within are believed to be effective. Because everyone is an individual and will respond differently to the use of essential oils, there is no guarantee as to the effectiveness or effects they will have on their use. No liability is taken for the implementation of the use of essential oils for any given person or persons.

The author has no control of the use of essential oils by others.

Table of Contents

Part ONE

Introduction
To
Aromatherapy

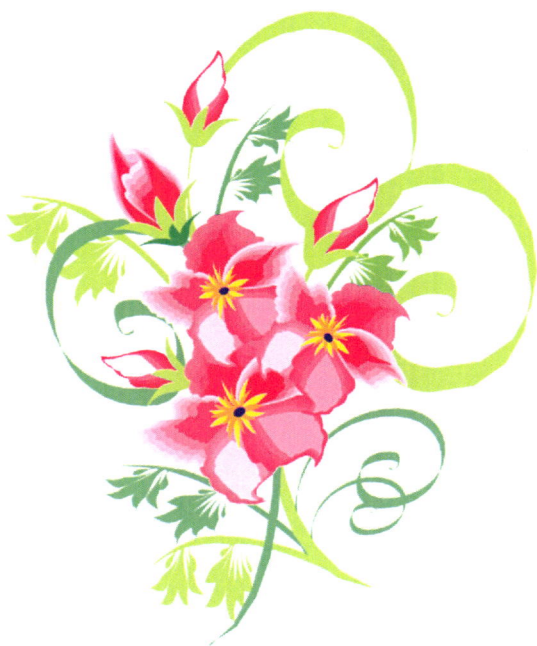

Introduction to Aromatherapy

What is Aromatherapy?

Aromatherapy means the study and use of scents as used in a **therapeutic** manner.

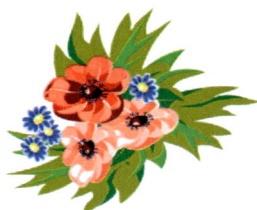

The more detailed definition is the skilled and controlled use of **essential oils** for emotional and physical health and well-being.

The practice of aromatherapy goes beyond smell, though. It involves "pure" essential oils and treatments many believe have a chemical effect on the body.

They can be applied with massage, in the bath or diffused into the air. They can be used in massage oils, lotions, hair care and many other applications.

Aromatherapy is a system of enabling the body to help heal itself by providing basic chemical constituents of the plants that the body may be missing or possibly out of balance.

What are essential oils?

Essential oils are the aromatic, subtle, volatile liquids that are distilled and extracted from plants and their parts: Flowers, Leaves, Berries, Seeds, Nuts, Roots, Bark, Twigs, Gums, Resins and Peels

An ancient process, essential oil distillation is a delicate and precise art that had almost been forgotten. Some oils are extracted by cold pressing such as the citrus oils. Others are extracted using carbon dioxide or other solvents.

Science is just now re-discovering the incredible healing power of essential oils, which some say are the life blood of the plant kingdom. Science and medicine are now beginning to acknowledge their value in physical and mental health care.

Most Essential oils have: Immune stimulating, Anti-viral, Anti-infectious, Anti-bacterial, Anti-microbial, Anti-septic, Anti-tumoral, Anti-fungal, and Anti-parasitic properties.

They can be Stimulating, Uplifting, Relaxing, Calming.
They can help with Memory, Focusing, Mental alertness.

Many folks use them while at work, at school, before and after sports, while meditating and much more.

The list is very large of the health concerns known to be helped with the use of essential oils.

Alternative or Complimentary?

Although listed as an Alternative Health modality, most Aromatherapists prefer to call it Complimentary Health care.

Aromatherapy should not be used to replace your regular health care, but as an addition to compliment your health care program and support your well being.

Please be sure to keep your Health Care Provider informed when you choose to use Essential oils and Aromatherapy as part of your health care regimen.

The Different Types of Aromatherapy

There are several ways to implement aromatherapy.

The kind this booklet is directed to is the practice of Holistic Therapeutic Aromatherapy. Holistic Aromatherapy involves looking at the body as a whole.

This means choosing the right essential oils to bring about the intended results for the physical and emotional well being of the persons seeking help.

Other types of Aromatherapy are practiced by Nursing Staff and Medical doctors, Esthetics, Psychological, Spirituality (essential oils are used throughout the world in religious and other ritual ceremonies) and for use with Animals.

But no matter what category of aromatherapy is practiced - they all use essential oils. And many of these types are interlinked with one another.

FUN FACTS

Did you know that it takes almost 2000 lbs – yep 1 ton of rose petals to make 1 pound (just about 2 cups) of Rose Otto – the essential oil of Rosa damascena?   That's one big field of flowers!!

In contrast, it only takes a few 100 pounds of Eucalyptus leaves to make several pounds of eucalyptus oil. (In production – essential oils are sold by the kilogram or pound).

A GLOBAL AFFAIR

Ever see those picture puzzles that show fields of flowers?
Guess what?   Those flowers are harvested and steam distilled to
get their essential oils.

Roses are mainly grown in Bulgaria, Turkey and a few other
countries. But Bulgaria and Turkey are known for the best Rose
Oils around the world!

Essential oils only come from plant sources and are sourced every
where from around the world.

Bulgaria – Lavender, Rose and many others
Turkey – Rose oil and Oregano oil
Australia – Eucalyptus oil and Tea Tree oil
India – Sandalwood oil
Madagascar – Jasmine and Ylang-ylang
Corsica – Helichrysum
England – Roman Chamomile and Lavenders
Italy – Bergamot, Lemon and Lime oils
USA – Peppermint and Grapefruit

The list goes on. Just about every county throughout the world
produce different essential oils.

This list is just a very tiny list of all the places around the world that
produce essential oils.

There are about 450 different essential oils that are used in
industry.   Only about 100 or so are used in Therapeutic
Aromatherapy.   Many of the others are used in the Perfumery and
Food and Flavoring industries.

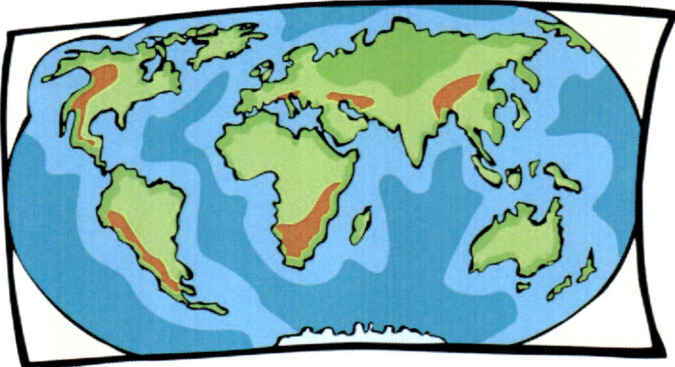

ESSENTIAL OIL SAFETY

This is a very important aspect of aromatherapy. Essential oils are very potent and highly concentrated chemicals extracted from plants by distillation.

One needs to remember that only a drop or two of essential oils are needed in most applications.

Some essential oils are more mild (Lavender) while others are extremely strong (Peppermint, Thyme and Oregano) when applied to the skin and also when inhaled. But just because an essential oil may have a light smell doesn't mean it won't have strong properties for emotional and health reasons.

Any essential oil can be a potential poison and so caution needs to be used around children, pets and the elderly. When using recipes for children and the elderly, cut the essential oil amounts in half but always use the normal amount of carrier oils in massage, lotion or other applications. And then when applied, use only small amounts on children and the elderly .

Please keep all essential oils out of the reach of children! And we don't mean just toddlers. Unless your teenager has been properly instructed, they too, should be using essential oils with adult supervision.

Some other major concerns are sensitization and skin irritations. A simple way to check to see if you have sensitive skin to any oil, you can test a small amount of essential oil (a drop diluted with carrier oil) on the inner arm (near the elbow). Observe for 24 hours, if no reaction, then you can proceed using on a routine basis. Of course, if at any time while using essential oils you see or feel an unpleasant reaction, discontinue use.

Any cold pressed or expressed citrus oil can cause a photo sensitivity reaction to occur. If applied to the skin and then exposed to sunlight or UV light such as in tanning salons, discoloration and burn can occur. Avoid using citrus essential oils or blends for several hours prior to exposure to either of these. Or use essential oils that have been stream distilled. In the case of Bergamot, use Bergamot FCF (Furo-coumarin Free) as this extraction of Bergamot is safe to use on skin should it be exposed to sunlight or UV rays.

What about using essential oils during pregnancy? Since most essential oils are found in everyday products like toothpaste, foods and household products many of them are also safe to use when pregnant. Although to be on the safe side, using essential oils for other applications and just like any other drug or strong chemical, it is suggested, that most essential oils be avoided during the first trimester.

After those first three months many essential oils can be used in moderation. Inhalation is preferred over skin applications. Again, when used in massage blends, follow the recommended recipe.

If the recipe pertains specifically to a pregnancy you can follow the recipe as written or if the recipe if for the general population, cut the essential oils in the recipe by half.

There is much controversy about using essential oils with those that have epilepsy or high blood pressure. Although there has not been much documentation done on essential oils causing problems with either. If you feel you should avoid certain essential oils, by all means, do so.

However, there is documentation that suggests strong odors or smells can sometimes trigger an epileptic seizure. If you are unsure one may want to avoid essential oils such as Eucalyptus globulus and Rosemary, other oils that may be included but are not limited to this list are Camphor and Tea Tree.

And before I forget, do not take essential oils internally. The term Aroma - Therapy, means to smell the aromas for therapy. It doesn't say to swallow them ever (unless prescribed by a medical doctor).

Herbs are made for ingesting not essential oils. And this book is about AROMA THERAPY not herbs!

Essential oils should always be diluted if applying to the skin. The old assumption that certain essential oils can be used directly (also known as "Neat or Neatly") on the skin should be revised.

Although Lavender and Tea Tree were once considered safe to use undiluted on the skin, just ask anyone that used to do so on a regular basis and now can **never** use those oils again due to the allergic reaction they have developed.

Only on rare occasions and only as a one time application should you ever apply Lavender or Tea Tree to the skin undiluted. A small drop on a wound or burn one time may not cause any problems but repeated applications of undiluted essential oils used while the wound heals could have unpleasant side effects down the road.

Do not apply essential oils diluted or not diluted to mucous membranes (eyes, mouth, vagina, rectum). Never apply to the eyes and use extreme caution if applying oils and lotions that contain essential oils near or around the eyes.

If you are unsure about using an essential oil, then don't use it.

Often times there are other essential oils that can be blended that can bring about the desired effect you are trying to achieve.

The main safety points are:

- Keep out of the reach of Children and Pets.
- Use essential oils sparingly. More is not better.
- Use half the amount on children and the elderly.
- Avoid using the photosensitive essential oils for several hours before going into the sun.
- Do not use undiluted on the skin, if in doubt do a skin test before using any oil.
- Do not ingest.
- Do not use essential oils during the first three months of Pregnancy, then limit thereafter, if you are concerned.
- Use caution with strong smelling oils around those with epilepsy.
- Avoid using essential oils around the eyes and other mucous membranes.
- Check with your medical practioner if you have any health concern and/or are taking prescription medicines.
- One special note about Cats and Essential oils. A cats liver cannot metabolize or break down most essential oils so if you own cats, use caution using essential oils around them. Never ever apply essential oils to your cat.

Essential oils are wonderful products of nature. When used safely, they will truly enhance your life and the lives of those around you. Enjoy!!

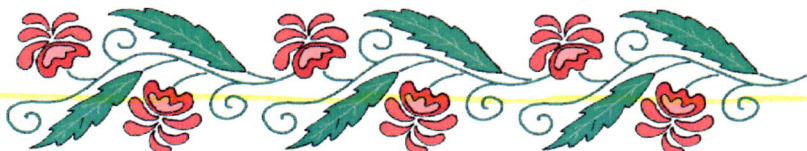

BLENDING AND MEASURING

When blending your essential oils remember to measure carefully. Most of the time you will be measuring drops of essential oils.

Almost all recipes are given by numbers of drops that are added. Many recipes are proportional - meaning that if a recipe calls for 5 drops of this oil, 3 drops of that oil, you can always mix 5 ml of this oil and 3 ml of that oil.

If you are trying to mix your essential oils with a water based product or in water. You may need to first mix it with an Emulsifier.

 An emulsifier is anything that will allow you to mix oil and water. Common products are coconut emulsifier, perfumers alcohol, Polysorbate 20, 60 or 80, turkey red castor oil to name a few. This will help the essential oils to blend with your water based products.

When mixing essential oils with carrier oils for use in massage you should never make a stronger blend than 2-3%.

How to figure out how much is in a 2% or 3% solution? First think of things in drops. If you have 100 drops of something you would have a 2 percent solution if 2 drops were an essential oil and 98 drops were a carrier oil. Or another way to measure it would be 2 ml of essential oil and 98 ml of the carrier oil.

Looking at the first example. 2 drops of Essential oil - that is easy. But the 98 drops of carrier oil that is not so easy, but you can do a little more math and convert the drops into teaspoons. Since there are about 20 drops per ml and 5 ml per teaspoon you can easily figure it out. 98 divided by 20 is approximated 5. So you have 5 ml or 1 teaspoon (or 98-100 drops of carrier oil).

A 2% solution would be 2 drops essential oil per teaspoon of carrier oil. 3% would be 3 drops per teaspoon.

Some essential oils work better when mixed with different carrier oils. So if you see your essential oils not mixing with particular carrier oil, you will have to experiment with another carrier oil.

Some essential oils and absolutes will become 'saturated' into a carrier oil. When this occurs you can not get any more essential oil or absolute to mix in with the carrier oil.

You will see it initially being in solution, but if you let it set for a day or two, you will either see the absolute sitting on the bottom, or the essential oil sitting on the top of your carrier oil.

Actually, this can happen with any unscented base product used. Shampoos, conditioners, and lotions are all prone to having the essential oil separate out. (Did you remember to use an emulsifier for your shampoo or bottle of water in your spray mister?)

Simply shake, or stir your bottle of product to mix the essential oils back into the product before using. Actually, shaking your blends a little before using is a good thing to do so as to redistribute your essential oils in the product.

There are a few essential oils when blended together that will not mix or they actually will cause a chemical reaction and become a solid chunk of 'goo' in the bottom of your bowl, bottle or jar. Fortunately, this is rare.

Do not let anything stop you from being creative. Essential oils are oils composed of several different chemical constituents. When mixed together you will sometimes see them get cloudy, then add another essential oil and the mixture will become clear. Sometimes the blend will cause sediment to form.

These are normal reactions when you mix certain essential oils together. Even though you are not a chemist you will eventually observe these reactions when blending different oils or when making up our blends.

Next: Store your custom blends of essential oils in glass bottles. Be sure to put labels on them with the essential oils you used. You will be able to use a drop or two without having to mix it fresh each time you want to enjoy your favorite blend. BUT only mix as much as you will use in 4-6 months. You always want to try to use the freshest blends and essential oils.

When mixing massage or bath blends we suggest you mix the essential oils together first before you add the carrier oil. Then let the mixture "age" or blend for several days before using.

Remember also that pure essential oils will disintegrate rubber and certain types of plastic materials. Never leave your bottles stopped with rubber bulb capped droppers. In just a few days the rubber

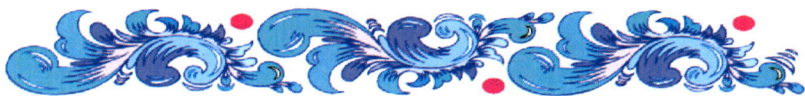

will be a terrible blob of black goo!

To blend essential oils with carrier oils you can mix them in PET plastic bottles or Glass bottles. PET plastic bottles will not deteriorate when used with essentials oils, other types of plastic bottles may.

MEASURING AND CONVERTING TO COMMON AMOUNTS

Blending essential oils and creating new scents can be fun. Writing down your measurements and quantities so you can use the same formulation again can be confusing.

So here are some common measurements to help guide you.

1 mL (milliliter) is equivalent to 20 –25 drops, The reason for the variable is related to two factors. One the thickness or viscosity of the essential oils and absolutes.   Drops can be larger than 'thin' oils. The other is the size of the opening of your dropper or pipette. You have to be consistent when writing your recipes, so be sure you indicate what type of dropper or pipette you were using. It can make a difference.

5 mL is 1 teaspoon
3 teaspoons is 1 tablespoon
2 tablespoons 1 ounce

Metric Measure	Decimal for fluid ounces	Common Fraction for fluid ounces	By drops (approximate due to viscosity of each essential oil)
1 mL	0.0335 fl oz	1 /30 fl oz	20-25
2 mL	0.067 fl oz	1/15 to 1/16 fl oz	40-50
4 mL	0.135 fl oz	1/8 (approximately) fl oz	80-100
5 mL	0.169 fl oz	1/6 fl oz	100-125
10 mL	0.33 fl oz	1/3 fl oz	Drops should not be
15 mL	0.5 fl oz	1/2 fl oz	counted for blending
29.573 mL	1 fl oz	1 fl oz	large amounts of
30 mL	1.014 fl oz	1 fl oz	essential oils therefore
50 mL	1.69 fl oz	1 2/3 fl oz	no drop values for these
60 mL	2 28 fl oz	2 fl oz	have been listed.

SUPPLIES FOR BLENDING

A good selection of the following items will make your blending experience more enjoyable.   Buying equipment and supplies you use just for your aromatherapy blending and storing them together makes it much easier for you to have fun and be creative.

- Small bottles for storing your blends such as:
  2ml, 4ml and 10 ml sizes with caps and orifice reducers
- Glass bottles in 1 and 2 ounce sizes.
- Several PET plastic bottles in 2, 4 or 8 ounce sizes.
- Caps for the plastic bottles—disc top and spray top
- Disposable pipettes or small glass dropper
- Beakers and Stirring Rods
- Glass Liquid Measuring cups (the kind with pouring spouts.)
- Stainless steel Measuring spoons and stirring spoons
- Wire Whip or French Whisks
- Larger Stainless Steel or Glass Mixing bowls (do not use plastic)
- Paper towels cut into quarters sheets (helpful when wiping up little messes).
- Electric hand mixer (may be helpful if mixing larger batches of lotions)
- Wax paper or freezer paper to cover your counter or table tops. Makes cleanup much quicker and protects your furniture finishes from being damages should any undiluted essential oils spill on them.

HELPFUL LIST of INGREDIENTS for use with this BOOK

(Essential oils will be listed on another page)

Now that you have read a little about aromatherapy you will want to experiment making some blends. Or maybe you have a health ailment you would like to help with a little massage.

Here is a list of ingredients used in this book. Always feel free to experiment with different carrier oils, lotions, creams, shampoos etc. You imagination and creativity are limited only by your own self.

- Sweet Almond Oil
- Apricot Kernel Oil
- Jojoba
- Sunflower Oil
- Grape seed Oil
- Aloe Vera
- Coconut oils
- Sesame Oil
- Emulsifier
- Distilled Water
- Lotions
- Sorbolene Cream

- Shampoo
- Conditioner
- Shower Gel
- Liquid Soap
- Body and Linen Spray
- Fan Type diffuser
- Tart or Oil Warmer
- Tea light diffuser
- Nasal Inhalers
- Aromatherapy Jewelry
- Terra Cotta diffusers

- Cotton balls
- Q-tips
- Silk Flowers
- Terry towels
- Water basins for hand foot soaks
- Potpourri
- Talc powder
- Baking soda
- Corn Starch

CLEANING YOUR GLASSWARE

After a busy day of blending or if you wish to reuse your essential oil bottles you will need to clean them thoroughly.

Use the hottest water available and some soap or detergent. Let them soak for a few minutes. Use a small bottle or baby nipple cleaning brush to clean the insides. Especially if you need to remove sediment. In tiny bottles you can use a Q-tip or tooth pick to remove stubborn remnants.

Rinse with more hot water, and turn upside down to drain on clean paper towels.

You are not done yet though, as you still could have a little bit of essential oil residue left inside your bottles or droppers.

The last thing to do is to rinse them with alcohol. We don't recommend rubbing or denatured alcohol as they have too much water content and other impurities in them. You can use a high "proof" cheap vodka. It is virtually odorless and has no impurities.

The alcohol dissolves and helps remove any residual essential or carrier oils that might be in your bottles and droppers.

Using alcohol as the final rinse will help your glassware to dry quickly, enabling you to be able to store them away for your next blending session.

Do not try to clean anything that is made of plastic as essential oils quickly permeate this and make it nearly impossible to remove scents.

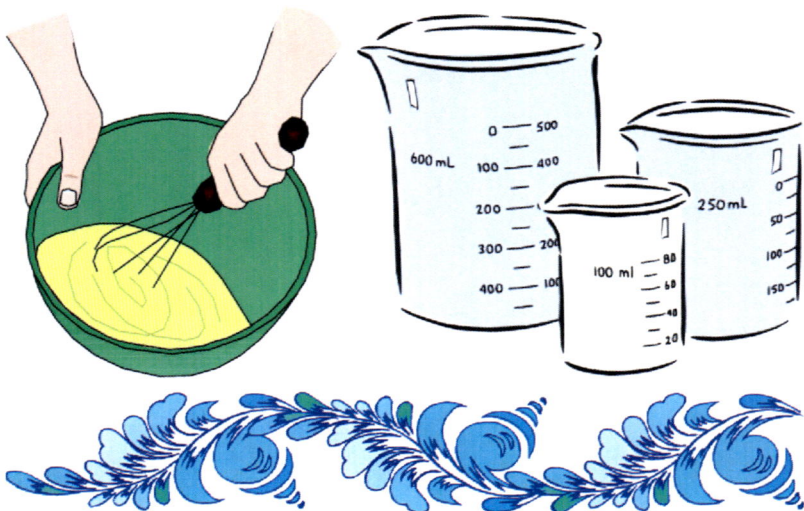

Ingredients for use with this book

ESSENTIALS OILS in this Book.

- Allspice
- Anise
- Basil
- Bay Laurel
- Bay Rum
- Bergamot
- Bergamot FCF
- Black Pepper
- Cajeput
- Carrot seed
- Cedarwood, Atlas
- Chamomile, German
- Chamomile, Roman
- Cinnamon Leaf
- Citronella
- Clary Sage
- Clove Bud
- Coriander
- Cypress
- Elemi
- Eucalyptus Globulus
- Eucalyptus Radiata
- Fennel
- Frankincense
- Geranium
- Ginger
- Grapefruit
- Helichrysum
- Hyssop
- Jasmine Absolute
- Juniper Berry
- Lavender, Bulgarian
- Lavender, French
- Lemon
- Lemongrass
- Lime
- Litsea cubeba (MayChang)
- Mandarin
- Marjoram, Sweet
- Melissa
- Myrrh
- Myrtle
- Naiouli
- Neroli
- Nutmeg
- Orange, Sweet
- Oregano
- Palmarosa
- Patchouli
- Peppermint
- Petitgrain
- Pine Needle
- Ravensara
- Rose Absolute
- Rose Otto
- Rosemary
- Rosewood
- Sage
- Sandalwood, India
- Spearmint
- Spruce Needle
- Tangerine
- Tea Tree
- Thyme
- Vanilla Absolute
- Vetiver
- Ylang-ylang

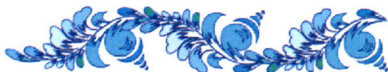

Remember many essential oils have similar properties and if you are short on one essential oil or don't have it—you might be able to find another essential oil or two you like better. Or you can just omit it this one time.

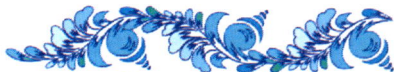

Essential Oil and Their Recipes have more than one use. Yes, Really They Do!

Mother Nature is so versatile and the plants and animals she provides us with have so many uses.

Just think about a tree for example. It can be used to build a home or furniture or eating utensils. It can be used for fuel to heat homes and businesses. And if left in it's natural state can provide shade in the summer and not to mention how lovely it looks in your yard or the forest.   Not to mention the flowers, leaves, twigs, bark and roots might be used to make those wonderful essential oils!

Essential oils are no different.   They have many different properties or uses. All are germicidal to varying degrees whether it be for viruses, bacteria or fungi.

Then they each possess a large variety of physical, emotional and spiritual properties. This helps them to be used in so many different applications.

So when you are looking for a recipe for a problem whether it be a illness or ailment, Be sure to use a good reference book that lists the various properties of essential oils too.

As an example, If you need a blend or recipe that has good decongestant properties and you know that Eucalyptus Globulus can do that really well.   Looking through this book you find a blend that has Eucalyptus Globulus . Even if the recipe title suggests it is for cleaning out the trash bin. That recipe may work great for your congestion!

Realize that the essential oils in that blend, although good for cleaning out the trash bin, also have some great essential oils to help with congestion. Blend it up and use it for congestion.

Also most all recipes can be easily adapted for use in other applications. An example here is: you find this great massage blend that you really love the smell of and would like to diffuse it in the bedroom.   Simply blend just the essential oils together in a glass bottle, omit the carrier oils or lotion and use in any diffuser.

Essential oil are so versatile and you being so creative can use many of these base recipes to have fun and a healthier and happier family and home.

Have fun, enjoy and most of all be creative!

NOTES

A Blank Page for you to Add your Own Notes. You will find areas like these occasionally entered, throughout this book. It will help you to keep track of your additions or changes to any recipe. Or you can Add your Own recipes as you would like.   Yep, Notes are good!

PART TWO

The Recipes
using
Pure Essential oils
and Absolutes.

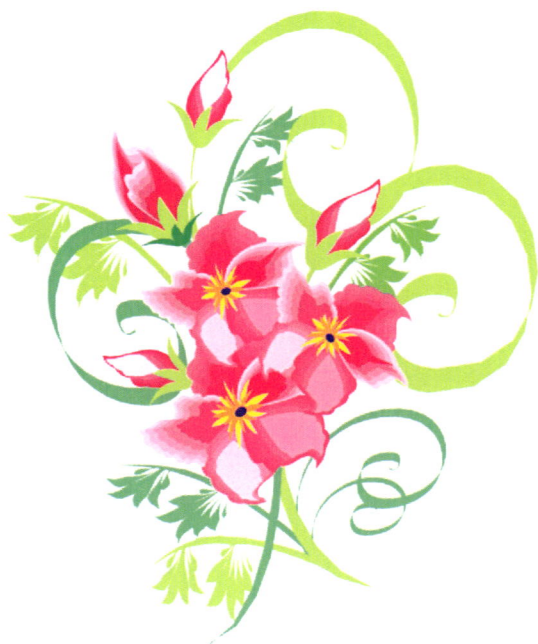

Happiness Blend
Orange 19 drops
Geranium 5 drops
Clove 1 drop
Cinnamon 1 drop
Rose Otto 1 drop

Blend all and diffuse. Or if you chose, place 5 drops into the bath.

Anxiety Diffuser Blend
Clary Sage 15 drops
Bergamot 10 drops
Geranium 10 drops
Chamomile 8 drops
Marjoram 8 drops
Ylang-ylang 5 drops

Blend the above essential oils in an glass bottle. Add some to a diffuser or smell from a drop applied to a cotton ball.

Penny's Favorite Blend
Grapefruit 10-15 drops
Spearmint 5-10 drops

This blend will often times smell like one of the Wrigley's chewing gums and is a very pleasant scent to use in any home or office. It is wonderful to stimulate and give you the pick me up you will need in the afternoon or any time of the day.

Serenity Blend
Sandalwood 20 drops
Jasmine 10 drops
Lavender 10 drops
Rosewood 10 drops
Roman Chamomile 5 drops
Neroli 5 drops

Blend all in an glass bottle. Then diffuse in any personal or room diffuser.

Enlivening Blend
Sweet Almond Oil 60 ml
Rosemary 10 drops
Peppermint 6 drops
Geranium 4 drops
Lemon 3 drops

Mix the essential oils, then add the carrier oil and mix well. Apply after or during a bath. This is an excellent blend for those experiencing Jet Lag.

Energize Me
Lavender 8 drops
Lemon 2 drops
Orange 6 drops
Rosemary 4 drops

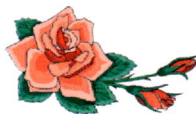

Blend these well in an glass bottle. Then diffuse in the air as needed, or use in a personal inhaler.

Fatigue Help
Spruce Needle 5 drops
Cedarwood 2 drops
Peppermint 1 drop

Mix the above together and use in a personal inhaler.

Concentration Blend
Lemon 20 drops
Basil 6 drops
Rosemary 2 drops

Mix oils, then diffuse into the air.

Concentration Blend #2
Orange 20 drops
Basil 10 drops
Rosemary 5 drops

Mix in an glass bottle. Then diffuse in any diffuser or smell directly from a personal inhaler.

Diffusion Blends and Sprays

Silk Flower Floral Scent
Vanilla 5 drops
Geranium 25 drops
Petitgrain 25 drops
Ylang-ylang 50 drops

Blend well in an
glass bottle then
apply a few drops to
several petals of a
silk flower
arrangement.
Reapply as desired.

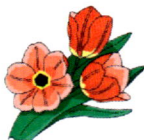

For Your Sprayer
(A Light Wonderful Air Freshener)
Lavender 15 drops
Orange 10 drops
Lemon 10 drops
Grapefruit 10 drops
Lime 6 drops
Nutmeg 3 drops
Distilled Water 2 ounces
Emulsifier 4-5 ml

Blend all the oils in a spray
bottle, add the emulsifier and
then the distilled water.
Shake well and spray.
This is an excellent air freshener
for pet odors.

We personally use this blend in
our home. It really is great when
mildew develops from high
humidity days.

Refreshing Mint Blend
Peppermint 5 drops
Lime 9 drops
Eucalyptus 1 drop

Blend well in a glass bottle, then
put in any diffuser.

Great for use in bathrooms or
other small rooms.

Spicy-Citrus Blend
Clove bud 6 drops
Lime 5 drops
Cinnamon 4 drops
Lemon 2 drops
Orange 2 drops

Blend all together and diffuse in
any room diffuser for your fall
room freshening and
disinfecting.

Spice Air Freshener
Rosemary 25 drops
Sage 25 drops
Spearmint 25 drops
Clove 25 drops
Patchouli 25 drops
Emulsifier 5 ml
Distilled Water 4 –6 ounces

Blend the essential oils with
Emulsifier, then add to
4 –6 ounces distilled water.
Shake well, then let sit for a day.
Spray in any room.

Spice Air Freshener #2
Anise 10 drops
Cinnamon Leaf 10 drops
Ginger 10 drops
Clove 15 drops
Orange 10 drops
Emulsifier 2 mls

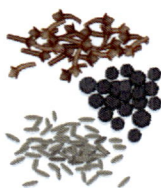

Blend the above
mixture in a
2 ounce glass spray top bottle.
Add purified or distilled water
and shake well.
Spray around the room as
desired.

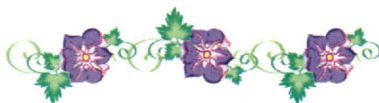

Joyful Spring Time Diffuser Blend

Orange 20 drops
Bergamot 20 drops
Basil 10 drops

Blend well in and glass bottle, then put several drops in any diffuser of your choice.

Way To Cool Down Spray

Clary Sage 4 drops
Roman Chamomile 3 drops
Geranium 3 drops
Cypress 2 drops
Peppermint 1 drop
Emulsifier—15-20 drops
Body Spray 8 ounces

Mix essential oils in bottle with the emulsifier and then add the body spray. Spritz yourself as needed to cool down.
Shake well before each use.
Keep refrigerated between uses .
(Discard after 30 days)

Clothes In The Cedar Closet Scent

Cedarwood Atlas 40 drops
Clove Bud 15 drops
Orange 15 drops

Blend in an glass bottle. Then put several drops on a Terra Cotta disc diffuser and let it soak in.

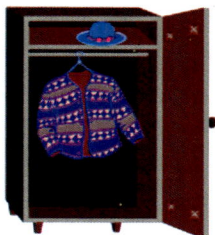

Then simply place in the corner or on a shelf in your closet. If you like the smell of cedarwood, this is a great blend for you.

Comforting Spray

Lavender 8 drops
Vanilla 3 drops
Ylang-ylang 3 drops
Orange 10 drops
Cedarwood 8 drops
Emulsifier 2 1/2 mL
Distilled Water 2 ounces

Add oils to emulsifier, shake well then add the distilled water. Shake well and spray in room.

Comforting Blend #2

Rose Otto 10 drops
Vanilla 3 drops
Roman Chamomile 3 drops
Mandarin 2 drops

Blend well in an glass bottle. Place a drop on a tissue and inhale.

This is a very strong blend. So if you choose to diffuse this place only 2-3 drops in your diffuser at a time. Adjust as necessary.

Odor Beater For Those Really Bad Smells!

Lemon 40 drops
Cinnamon Leaf 40 drops
Peppermint 40 drops
Lemongrass 25 drops
Emulsifier 2 teaspoons
Distilled Water 4 ounces

Blend the essential oils with the emulsifier. Shake and blend well. Then add the 4 ounces of distilled water.
Shake well before each use, spray as needed in the odoriferous room.

This mixture will be cloudy.

Refreshing Spray
Distilled Water 8 ounces
Lime 90 drops
Peppermint 50 drops
Eucalyptus 10 drops
Emulsifier 10 ml

Add the essential oils and the
emulsifier into a clean bottle
then pour the distilled water
into the bottle. Shake well then
spray in the air.
Shake well before each use.

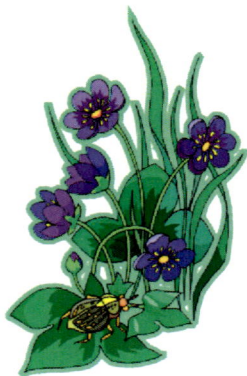

Citrus Surprise
Lime 50 drops
Grapefruit 50 drops
Orange 10 drops
Patchouli 10 drops
Emulsifier 5 mls
Distilled water 4 ounces

Place the essential oils and
emulsifier in a clean spray bottle,
then the distilled water into the
bottle. Shake well before each
use.

The above 2 blends can be used
in any diffuser. Just blend the
essential oils in an glass bottle,
shake well put a few drops in
your diffuser

Spray Air Freshener
Marjoram 25 drops
Sage 25 drops
Spearmint 25 drops
Clove Bud 25 drops
Patchouli 20 drops
Distilled Water 4 ounces

Mix all oils and add to the
distilled water. Shake well and
use in a sprayer.
Shake well before each use.

Room Fragrance
Lime 80 drops
Bergamot 60 drops
Tangerine 30 drops
Petitgrain 15 drops
Patchouli 10 drops
Emulsifier 2 teaspoon
Distilled Water 4-6 ounces

Mix the essential oils with
emulsifier, then add the distilled
water. Use in a spray bottle.
Shake well before each use.

This blend may be cloudy, this is
normal.

When Entertaining
Bergamot 3 drops
Geranium 2 drops
Lavender 3 drops

Use the above essential oils
blend in a tea light diffuser or a
fan diffuser while entertaining.

This blend gives off a wonderful
atmosphere when friends are
gathered together.

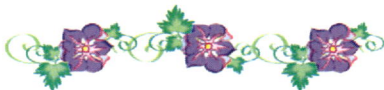

Entertaining Diffuser Blend

Bergamot 3 drops
Geranium 2 drops
Lavender 3 drops

Use the above essential oils blend in a Scentball diffuser, tea light diffuser or a fan diffuser while entertaining.

This blend gives a wonderful atmosphere when friends are gathered together.

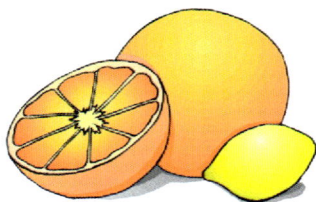

Citrus Scent For Any room

Lemon 10 drops
Lime 5 drops
Tangerine 4 drops
Mandarin 3 drops
Patchouli 3 drops

Blend all in an glass bottle, then use in any room diffuser of your choice. Tea light or electric warmers are ideal for this room scent.

Citrus Air Freshener

Orange 10 drops
Lemon 10 drops
Grapefruit 10 drops
Cedarwood 5 drops
Cinnamon 3 drops

Blend this in an glass bottle and apply a few drops to your favorite diffuser.

Citrus Room Freshener

Orange 50 drops
Lemon 35 drops
Grapefruit 20 drops
Spearmint 20 drops
Sandalwood 15 drops
Emulsifier 1/2 teaspoon
Distilled Water 8 ounces
8oz PET plastic bottle with spray

Blend essential oils well in PET plastic bottle then add 1/2 teaspoon emulsifier. Mix thoroughly. Then add the distilled water and shake well. Spray around the room.

Keep unused spray in the refrigerator for future use! This room freshener can be used for any time. Light refreshing and a little sweet.

Citrus-Mint Body Spray

Orange 10 drops
Mandarin 10 drops
Lemon 6 drops
Grapefruit 6 drops
Peppermint 5 drops

Blend essential oils together in an glass bottle. Next in an 8 ounce PET bottle put 2mls of emulsifier then add the essential oils. Shake very well.

Then add 2 ounces of white vinegar and shake well. Fill the rest of the bottle with distilled water. Shake well before use.

Splash this on after your shower. It is very invigorating and should help energize you throughout your day.

Fresh and Fruity Hair Spray

Orange 15 drops
Neroli 12 drops
Emulsifier 25 drops
Distilled Water 2 ounces

Blend the essential oils and emulsifier in a 2 ounce PET plastic spray bottle the add the distilled water. Shake well before spraying on hair.

You can substitute a unscented body spray or hair de-tangler for the 2 ounces of distilled water.

Spring Floral Scent

Rosewood 10 drops
Ylang-ylang 10drops
Lemon 6 drops
Clove 6 drops
Cedarwood 4 drops

Mix the above essential oils in an glass bottle. Add some to any diffuser or drop inside the cardboard potion of the toilet paper roll to add scent to your bathroom.

Or add to the petals of the silk flower arrangement that sits in your bathroom.

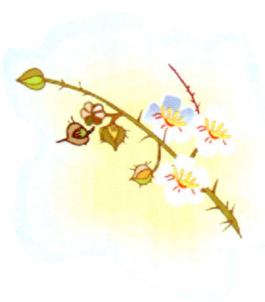

Floral Aromatic Water Spray

Ylang-ylang 50 drops
Geranium 25 drops
Petitgrain 25 drops
Vanilla 20 drops
Emulsifier 5 ml
Distilled water 8 ounces

Blend and shake well in a glass bottle. Let sit for a couple of weeks. Strain in a coffee filter or cheese cloth. Use to spray any room, linen etc.
You can use this blend as soon as you have mixed it, but it will improve with age.

Floral Springtime Room Spray

Orange 50 drops
Clove 20 drops
Cinnamon 15 drops
Jasmine 10 drops
Rose Otto 1 drop
Emulsifier 5 mL
Distilled Water 4 ounces

Blend the essential oils in a PET bottle, add the emulsifier and blend well some more. Then add the Distilled water, shake well until well blended. Just spray once or twice in a room.

Spicy Spray Bottle Blend

Orange 40 drops
Clove 30 drops
Bergamot 10 drops
Ginger 5 drops
Cinnamon 5 drops
Lemon 5 drops
Nutmeg 5 drops
Emulsifier 5 ml

Blend oils with emulsifier and add to 4-6 ounces distilled water. Shake well, then spray.

For Your Spray Bottle

Citronella 2 drops
Bergamot 2 drops
Frankincense 2 drops
Lemon 2 drops
Lavender 4 drops
Distilled Water 2 ounces

Pour blend into bottle, shake well and mist into your home. Caution – DO NOT spray onto furniture.

Comforting Spray

Lavender 8 drops
Vanilla 3 drops
Ylang-ylang 3 drops
Orange 10 drops
Cedarwood 8 drops
Emulsifier 1/2 teaspoon
Distilled Water 2 ounces

Add oils to emulsifier, shake well then add the distilled water. Shake well and spray in room.

Calming Mist Spray

Marjoram 30 drops
Cajeput 30 drops
Lavender 30 drops
Petitgrain 30 drops
Vetiver 30 drops
Emulsifier 10 ml
Pure Water 4-6 ounces

Mix together and spray in the room. This also works on overactive kids. Spray in evening and before bed to help them sleep.

Just So You Know!
Always keep your bottles of essential oils tightly capped. Oxygen can destroy and deteriorate your precious oils. Keep them cool too!

Calming Diffuser Blend

Roman chamomile 20 drops
Lavender 15 drops
Clary Sage 10 drops
Geranium 10 drops
Ylang-ylang 5 drops

Blend essential oils in a glass bottle and add to diffuser as needed.

Simple Stress Reducer Diffuser Blend

Sandalwood 10 drops
Lavender 5 drops
Spruce 5 drops
Rose absolute 1 drop

Blend in an glass bottle. Then diffuse in the room.

Refreshing Stress Blend

Lemon 10 drops
Lavender 15 drops
Clary Sage 5 drops

Blend in an glass bottle and diffuse. Can be used in a personal diffuser or any fan diffuser. This blend is also nice in the bath, about 5 drops will do.

Stimulating Living room Diffuser Blend

Grapefruit 8 drops
Lavender 4 drops
Lemon 4 drops
Basil 2 drops

Blend together in an glass bottle and place in your favorite diffuser. Start with just a few drops then add more as needed throughout the evening of entertaining.

Reduce Stress Diffuser Blend
Lavender 10 drops
Mandarin 10 drops

Blend and diffuse using a fan
diffuser or use in a personal
inhaler

A Little Spice Is Nice
(Refreshing Blend)
Orange 10 drops
Grapefruit 8 drops
Bergamot 4 drops
Ginger 4 drops
Clove Bud 4 drops
Cinnamon Leaf 3 drops

Blend all essential oils together
and diffuse in the air. Any
diffuser will work, but a tea light
diffuser will give a special
warmth to the enjoyment of the
spices in this blend.

Stimulating Personal Blend
Orange 6 drops
Clary sage 4 drops
Coriander 4 drops
Helichrysum 2 drop
Jasmine 2 drop
Palmarosa 2 drop
Vetiver 2 drop
Jojoba 1 ounce

Blend all in an glass bottle.
Wear as a fragrance or smell
directly from the bottle.

Contentment Diffuser Blend
Bergamot 10 drops
Clove 5 drops
Sandalwood 10 drops
Ylang-ylang 5 drops

Mix together and diffuse.
This blend can also be used to
settle restlessness.

Jitters Blend
Peppermint 5 drops
Spearmint 5 drops
Basil 2 drops

For jitters when attending
summer weddings, parties or
other gatherings where
strangers may be present.
This blend helps to gives you
courage to start conversations!
Place in a personal inhaler or
use on a tissue.

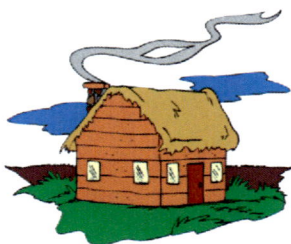

Cabin Fever
(Mild Depression)
Coriander 12 drops
Lemon 6 drops
Neroli 6 drops
Ylang-ylang 5 drops
Sunflower oil 1 ounce

Blend the above together.
Use up to a teaspoon of this
blend in a bath.

For Those LONG Winter Nights
(This is a great relaxer and soother)
Grapefruit 6 drops
Bergamot 6 drops
Lime 6 drops
Ginger 4 drops
Sandalwood 2 drops

Blend all oils and use in diffuser
or atomizer or place 5-6 drops in
your bath.

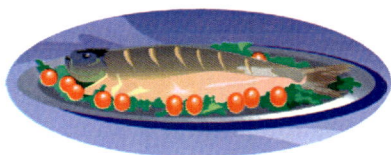

After The Fish Has Been Cooked Room Freshener

Lemon 20 drops
Bergamot 10 drops
Grapefruit 10 drops
Emulsifier 1/4 teaspoon
Distilled water 8 ounces
PET bottle with spray top

Blend essential oils well in PET plastic bottle, then add 1/4 teaspoon emulsifier. Mix thoroughly. Then add the distilled water and shake well. Spray around the room.

Relax and Wind Down Spray Mist

Mandarin 10 drops
Lavender 5 drops
Marjoram 3 drops
Sandalwood 3 drops
Emulsifier 25 drops
Distilled Water 4 ounces

Blend all essential oils together then add the emulsifier. Blend this well. Add the essential oils and emulsifier to a 4 ounce PET plastic spray bottle, add 4 ounces of distilled water. Shake well before each use.

This blend is great when your children need to wind down after an exciting day, such as a birthday party or when company comes to visit after dinner.

The Forest Scent

Spruce 10 drops
Lavender 3 drops
Clove Bud 3 drops
Rosemary 3 drops
Patchouli 1 drop

Blend all together and use in any diffuser.

Wonderful Summer Body Spray

Ylang -Ylang Extra 10 drops
Sandalwood 10 drops
Vanilla 4 drops
Litsea Cubeba 5 drops
Emulsifier 30 drops
Unscented Body Spray or
Distilled water 2 ounces

In a 2 ounce PET bottle, blend the essential oils together and add the emulsifier to this. Then add 2 ounces of unscented body spray. Shake well.

Spray on your body after showering or bathing, or any time you feel you want to freshen up your scent!

Mint Aromatic Water Spray

Peppermint 50 drops
Spearmint 50 drops
Patchouli 20 drops
Coconut emulsifier 5 mls
Distilled Water 4 ounces

Blend and shake well in a glass bottle. Let sit for a couple weeks.

Mix with emulsifier and then add the 4 ounces of distilled water, shake well.

You can use this blend as soon as you have mixed it, but will improve with age.

Minted Scents

Peppermint 10 drops
Rosemary 3 drops
Grapefruit 3 drops
Vanilla 1 drop

Blend all together and use in any diffuser.

.Acceptance Blend

Lavender 10 drops
Orange 10 drops
Cypress 5 drops
Roman Chamomile 5 drops

Blend all in an glass bottle. Then diffuse in any room diffuser.

Fatigue Relief Diffuser Blend

Peppermint 6 drops
Spearmint 6 drops
Rosemary 6 drops
Grapefruit 5 drops
Lemon 5 drops

Blend all ingredients in an glass bottle. Shake well to mix.

Then place in your favorite diffuser. Can also be used in a personal inhaler.

For Your Bath
Refreshing and Relaxing Oils

Fir 4 drops
Geranium 4 drops
Spearmint 4 drops
Juniper Berry 2 drops
Lemon 2 drops
Carrier oil 1 teaspoon

Mix well and add to a tub of very warm water and RELAX!!

Happy Bath Blend

Ylang-ylang 5 drops
Sandalwood 5 drops
Grapefruit 5 drops
Peppermint 1 drop

Mix all oils together in an glass bottle. Add several drops to your bath.

Calm the Jitters Bath Blend

Roman Chamomile 4 drops
Clary Sage 4 drops
Neroli 1 drop
Vetiver 1 drop

Add all to a warm tub, sit, soak, and relax. Light a candle or two and play some soothing music. Take some time to yourself.

Relaxing Hot Tub Blend
(For 4-5 People)

Spruce needle 5 drops
Vanilla 4 drops
Lemongrass 4 drops
Cedarwood 2 drops
Emulsifier 1 ml

Blend all in a PET plastic bottle then add about half to your hot tub. Add the remaining amount after 30 minutes, if desired.

Warming Winter Bath

Sandalwood 4 drops
Myrrh 4 drops
Ginger 4 drops
Whole Milk 1 cup

Add the essential oils to the milk, blend well. Then add to your tub. Relax.

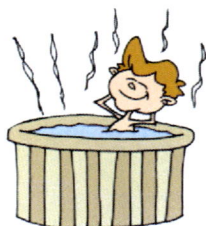

Relaxation Bath Blend
Lavender 3 drops
Basil 2 drops
Marjoram 2 drops
Fennel 1 drop
Vetiver 1 drop

Add to a warm bath, soak for
10 minutes or more.
Repeat as needed!!

Quiet Moments
Sandalwood 6 drops
Cedarwood 4 drops
Ylang-ylang 3 drops
Lavender 3 drops

Blend in a glass bottle. Add 8
drops to your bath water as it is
filling the tub.

Add a cup of Epsom salts or
baking soda or a combination to
help you have a very relaxing
and soothing bath.

Soak for 20-30 minutes adding
more hot water as desired.

(This blend makes enough for
two baths.)

Hemorrhoid Sitz Bath
Cypress 2 drops
Juniper berry 2 drops
Helichrysum 2 drops

Fill bath tub to hip deep (while
sitting in the tub).

Then add the above essential
oils, swish around. Then sit in
the warm bath for up to
20 minutes.

Increase Circulation Bath Blend
Cypress 2 drops
Juniper berry 2 drops
Peppermint 2 drops
Pine 2 drops
Rosemary 2 drops

Add the oils to a bathtub filled
with warm water. Soak and
Enjoy!

Foot Bath Rejuvenator
Myrtle 4 drops
Spearmint 4 drops
Grapefruit 4 drops
Cajeput 3 drops
Sweet Almond oil 5 ml

Blend together and add 7-9
drops in foot bath, swirl water to
disperse the oils, insert feet and
relax for 15 minutes.

Soaking Feet Blend to warm your whole body!
Lemon 10 drops
Geranium 6 drops
Rosemary 4 drops

Blend these in an glass bottle.
Then add 3-4 drops to a basin of
hot water, large enough to soak
your feet comfortably. Or place
up to 10 drops in a full tub of
water.

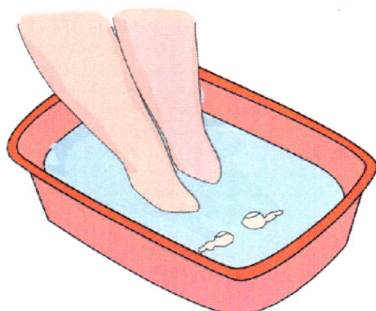

Refreshing Foot Bath
Rosemary 6 drops
Lavender 4 drops
Peppermint 2 drops
Tea Tree 1 drop

Fill a basin with warm water. Add essential oils. Soak your feet and enjoy. Soak for 10-15 minutes, adding more warm water if desired.

Swollen Feet Relief
Lavender 2 drops
Lemon 1 drop
Geranium 1 drop

Add the above essential oils to a basin of cool water.

Then soak a towel in the basin, wring out excessive water and wrap loosely around swollen feet and hands.

Elevate your feet and relax.

Be sure you have placed another towel to protect your pillows and furniture form becoming dampened.

Rest for 15-20 minutes as needed.

Brighten Me Bath Blend
Rosewood 5 drops
Palmarosa 5 drops
Grapefruit 5 drops
Petitgrain 2 drops
Jojoba 1 teaspoon

Fill the bath tub with warm water, add the above mixture to the tub and swish around.

If You Love Roses Bath
Rosewood 3 drops
Geranium 2 drops
Rose Absolute 1 drop

Add to a warm bath, float rose petals on top. Light a candle, play some soothing music and let you mind wander. Then simply enjoy!

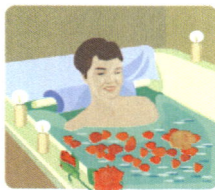

For A Quick Summer Time Hot Tub Or Bath Blend
Lavender 4 drops
Eucalyptus 4 drops
Juniper Berry 2 drops
Vanilla 2 drops

Blend together in an glass bottle. Then add the entire contents to your tub.

If you are using this blend in a very large hot tub, you will need to double this recipe for a four person tub.

Energizing Blend For The Hot Tub
Peppermint 20 drops
Lavender 20 drops
Cedarwood 20 drops
Spruce Needle 10 drops
Eucalyptus globulus 10 drops
Coconut emulsifier 1 teaspoon

Blend in a PET plastic bottle then add 3-4 drops per person to the hot tub. Add more if desired after 30 minutes.

Makes enough for several uses.

Tantalizing Bath

Patchouli 1 drop
Rose Otto 1 drop
Bergamot FCF 2 drops

Blend in a nice warm
Bath and enjoy.

The Tranquil Bath

Marjoram 3 drops
French Lavender 2 drops
Geranium 1 drop
Rose otto 1 drop
Jojoba 1teaspoon

Add all to your bath tub.
The wonderful relaxing and
mind replenishing properties
of these oils will be very
welcoming after a hectic day
of work or playing with the
kids.
The Jojoba will soften and
enhance your natural beauty.

Fight The Winter Blahs Bath

Orange 6 drops
Geranium 2 drops
Jojoba 1 teaspoon

Fill the tub with comfortably
warm water. Add the essential
oils, Jojoba and a few thin
slices of fresh cut orange.
Enjoy!

Stress Reducing Bath

Roman Chamomile 2 drops
Lavender 2 drops
Cypress 1 drop
Fennel 1 drop
Ginger 1 drop
Vetiver 1 drop

Add to your bathtub with
warm water and enjoy a
leisure soak for 20-30 minutes.

Stress Relieving—Muscle Relaxing Bath Tub Blend

Sandalwood 5 drops
Fennel 3 drops
Melissa 3 drops
Basil 2 drops
Lavender 2 drops

Also add 1-2 cups Epsom salts to
the tub while filling.

Epsom salts will help to relieve
tense muscles and make you feel
even more
relaxed.

Relaxing Bath

Lavender 6 drops
Roman chamomile 4 drops
Rosewood 4 drops
Vanilla absolute 2 drops
Neroli 2 drops
Rose 1 drop
Ylang-ylang 1 drop

Mix all in an glass bottle. This
recipe will make enough for 3-4
baths. As you will add about 5-6
drops to the tub of warm water
for each bath.

A De-Stressing Bath

Lavender 3 drops
Ylang-ylang 3 drops
Basil 2 drops
Geranium 2 drops
Grapefruit 2 drops

Fill the tub with warm
water, add the essen-
tial oils. Close the bath
room door, relax and
enjoy.

Light a few candles, play your favorite relaxing music and unwind.

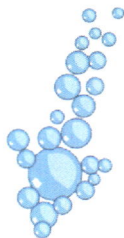

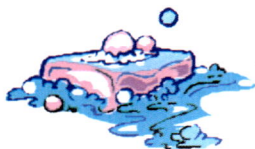

Stimulating Bath
When You Are On The Go!
Rosemary 6 drops
Juniper Berry 3 drops
Almond Oil 1 teaspoon

Add all to your bath tub.

Float a few dried flower petals on top of the water if desired.

This blend can also be used in the shower-for a pick me up in the morning. Omit the Sweet Almond Oil. Simply apply the essential oil drops to a terra cotta disc and let the essential oils soak into the disc.

Place in the corner of the shower where the water will hit it. It should wake you up and help you concentrate throughout the day.

Bath Oil For ADD/ADHD
Lavender 40 drops
Roman Chamomile 40 drops
Mandarin 60 drops
Sunflower Oil 1 teaspoon

Mix together in a PET bottle then add only 3 drops to the bath tub, no more. Swish around, let the child enjoy the tub for 10-20 minutes.

The small amount of carrier oil in this recipe should not make the tub or child slippery, but be aware that carrier oils in the bath tub can leave a r bath tub ring and could make it slippery.

Eliminating Toxins Bath
Oregano 6 drops
Juniper Berry 6 drops
Lemon 10 drops
Grapefruit 10 drops
Basil 8 drops

Blend the above essential oils in an glass bottle. Add only about 8 drops to the bath.

You can also add a cup of Epsom salts or other salts such as dead sea salts to the bath as well. While in the tub, massage (towards your heart– from toes to hips) the affected areas. This will help your body to eliminate toxins. Also be sure to drink plenty of water, before and after your bath. Don't forget to sit and soak for a few minutes.

Detoxifying Weekly
Bath Blend
Geranium 2 drops
Rosemary 2 drops
Juniper Berry 2 drops
Lavender 2 drops

Mix together in an glass bottle. Then add 5-8 drops to the bath. Also add 1-2 cups Epsom Salts. You might want to mix a larger quantity so you can use this on a weekly basis.

Relaxing Bath
Chamomile 4 drops
Lavender 2 drops

Put in a warm bath before bed as this is a relaxing blend.

Tense Neck Muscles
Lavender 8 drops
Lemon 4 drops
Peppermint 3 drops
Carrier oil of your choice 1
ounce

Sweet Almond and Sunflower
are wonderful for this blend.

Mix together in a plastic PET
bottle. Massage as needed on
the sore and tense neck
muscles.

Aches And Pains Rub
Oregano 3 drops
Peppermint 4 drops
Cedarwood 2 drops
Lavender 2 drops
Sweet Almond oil 1 tablespoon

Add essential oils to the
1 tablespoon almond oil. Stir or
shake well.

Massage into and rub out the
aches and pains.

Just So You Know!
Did you know that when you
massage an essential oil blend
on to your skin you might
taste it 20– 30 minutes later?

Your skin is the largest organ
of your body. Essential oil
molecules, being as small as
they are, can penetrate the
skin and send it's healing
properties to the area of the
body where the help is
needed.

Even a small amount of
essential oils can be
distributed throughout the
body in a few minutes.

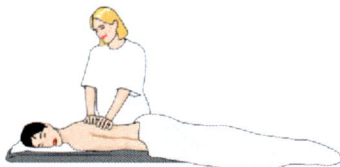

Your Next Relaxing Massage
Orange 4 drops
Anise 3 drops
Cedarwood 3 drops
Neroli 3 drops
Roman Chamomile 2 drops
Sunflower oil 1 tablespoon

Blend essential oils together and
add to sunflower oil, use for a
relaxing massage.

If you have Overworked Your Back
Lavender 10 drops
Rosemary 6 drops
Sandalwood 6 drops
Geranium 3 drops
Sweet Almond 1 ounce

Place the essential oils in an
glass bottle. Mix well. Add the 2
tablespoons of carrier oil. Shake
gently to mix well. Place a small
amount to the area of the back
that has discomfort.

This can also be applied prior to
strenuous activity or after you've
over done it.

Rubbing Oil for Sore Joints
Marjoram 10 drops
Eucalyptus 8 drops
Cajeput 4 drops
Black Pepper 2 drops
Carrier oil 2 ounces

Mix all oils and add to the carrier
oil. Shake well and warm gently
before massaging on sore joints.

.After a Hectic and Crazy Day Massage

Anise 6 drops
Nutmeg 6 drops
Rose Otto 1 drop
Carrier oil 2 ounces

Massage into upper chest, back of neck, across shoulders and mid back. Use it to relieve stress and is calming.

No Time For A Soak Massage Lotion?

Try the following blend mixed in lotion or a light carrier oil such as Sunflower.
Lavender 12 drops
Cypress 5 drops
Lemongrass 4 drops
Grapefruit 4 drops

Mix in 2 tablespoons lotion or oil. Apply a small amount to you legs and massage with strokes going towards your heart.

This will encourage proper blood drainage and will help to decrease swelling.

You can use this daily. Lotions will absorb more readily and make dressing easier after applying.

Muscle Relaxer Massage

Niaouli 20 drops
Lavender 15 drops
Black Pepper 12 drops
Pine 12 drops
Sunflower oil 2 ounces

Mix essential oils in a PET bottle then add carrier oil. Warm slightly and use for massage.

Penetrating Pain Relieving Massage Oil

Peppermint 5 drops
Allspice 5 drops
Marjoram 5 drops
Apricot oil 1 tablespoon

Blend all in a PET bottle, shake well. Massage into those painful spots.

Quick Relief Massage

Ginger 5 drops
Bay Laurel 5 drops
Marjoram 5 drops
Sunflower oil 1 tablespoon

Blend all together and use for massaging that back ache.

Relief For Tired Muscles

Spearmint 10 drops
Pine needle 6 drops
Ginger 4 drops
Black Pepper 4 drops
Sweet Almond 1 ounce

Blend well in a PET bottle. Shake well before using. Massage just a few drops into sore, tired muscles.

This may be a very warming massage blend.

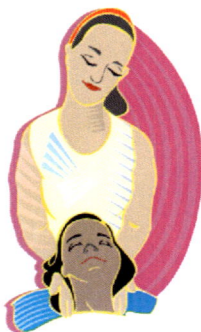

For General Joint Pains
Cypress 10 drops
Eucalyptus 9 drops
Ginger 6 drops
Hyssop 5 drops
Carrier Oil 1 ounce

Blend essential oils well into your favorite carrier oil or lotion. Massage onto affected joints 4-6 times a day. After 3 days, you can begin to apply heat compresses.

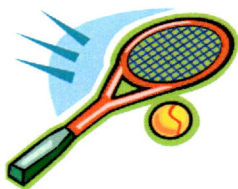

Tennis Elbow Massage
Eucalyptus 10 drops
Peppermint 5 drops
Ginger 10 drops
Rosemary 5 drops
Sunflower oil 1 ounce

Blend all in a bottle. Use to massage the affected forearm/ elbow area as needed.

A Foot Lotion For Painful Feet
Lavender 25 drops
Peppermint 10 drops
Eucalyptus 5 drops
Lotion base 2 ounces

Blend well and apply to clean feet several times a day as desired.

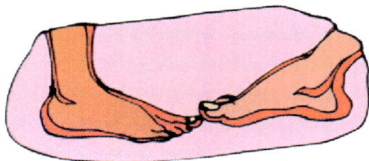

Warming Massage Blend
(Especially good for
sore joints as in arthritis)
Roman Chamomile 6 drops
Marjoram 8 drops
Coriander 6 drops
Rosemary 6 drops
Vanilla 2 drops
Black Pepper 2 drop
Ginger 2 drop
Carrier Oil 2 ounces

Blend well in a PET bottle. Massage daily into legs, knees or other sore joints.

 This blend will also work well to warm muscles before working out exercising.

Relaxing Massage #1
Lavender 10 drops
Mandarin 6 drops
Marjoram 6 drops
Roman Chamomile 6 drops
Sage 3 drops
Sweet Almond oil 2 ounces

Blend all essential oils in a PET plastic bottle, add the Sweet Almond oil. Shake well.

Use for massage especially on days where you are more stressed.

Relaxing Massage #2
Orange 4 drops
Anise 3 drops
Cedarwood 3 drops
Sandalwood 2 drops
Neroli 3 drops
Chamomile 2 drops
Sweet Almond 1 tablespoon

Blend well in a PET bottle and use for a relaxing massage.

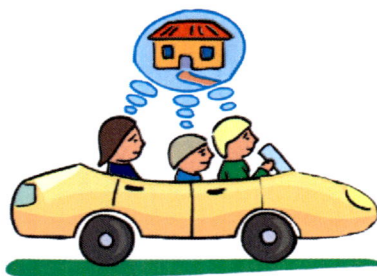

Drive, Drive, Drive
Massage Blend
Bay laurel 15 drops
Peppermint 12 drops
Roman Chamomile 12 drops
Juniper Berry 12 drops
Geranium 12 drops
Ginger 9 drops
Sweet Almond 2 ounces

Blend together in a PET bottle, shake well.

Have someone massage your upper back, shoulders, neck and lower back before and/or after a long day of driving to help relieve tense muscles.

Attentive Massage Blend
Peppermint 5 drops
Clove Bud 5 drops
Thyme 5 drops
Carrier oil 1 tablespoon

Blend well and let sit for one day, then use as you would any other massage blend.

This oils in this blend will also help with cold and flu.

 Rub on the bottom of your feet if you are feeling a little under the weather.

For The Car Ride Home
Rosemary 5 drops
Lime 4 drops
Bergamot 6 drops

Blend all of these in a small glass bottle. Then apply 2-4 drops on pad of your electric car diffuser. If using a terra cotta diffuser you may want to add several drops.

This recipe will also work great to help any student stay awake and alert while studying.

Energize Me Massage Oil
Lavender 6 drops
Rosemary 4 drops
Geranium 3 drops
Lemongrass 3 drops
Coriander 2 drops
Patchouli 2 drops
Sunflower 2 ounces

Blend essential oils in a PET bottle, then add the sunflower oil. Mix well and massage into your skin as desired.

Uplifting Massage
Spearmint 5 drops
Basil 3 drops
Lime 3 drops
Rosemary 3 drops
Eucalyptus 3 drops
Bergamot 3 drops
Carrier Oil 20 mls

Add essential oils to a 1 ounce glass bottle, then add carrier oil. Mix well and use for massage.

Omit the carrier oil and use this blend in any diffuser.
It is wonderfully refreshing.

Digestive Stimulant
Bergamot FCF 5 drops
Ginger 3 drops
Roman Chamomile 3 drops
Grape seed oil 1 ounce

Blend the oils and massage
stomach and intestinal area in
a clockwise direction using
small circular movements.

For A Back Ache Massage
Lavender 10 drops
Rosemary 6 drops
Sandalwood 6 drops
Geranium 3 drops
Almond Oil 1 ounce

Mix in an glass bottle, shake
well and apply to areas of
discomfort.

"Oh My Aching Back" Massage
Lavender 20 drops
Rosemary 15 drops
Peppermint 5 drops
Eucalyptus 5 drops
Almond Oil 2 ounces

Blend all essential oils in a PET
bottle, add almond oil.
Shake well. Have someone give
you a 10-15 minute massage
on those sore back muscles
and other areas.

Relief For Sore Fatigued Back Muscles
Peppermint 5 drops
Eucalyptus globulus 5 drops
Lavender 5 drops
Almond Oil 1 tablespoon

Blend well in a PET bottle.
Shake well before massaging
into sore back muscles.

Helpful Hint
Gently heat massage oil before
using. Your recipient of the
massage will love the feeling of
warmed oils when applied to
the skin. And it will excite the
essential oils molecules and help
them to enter the room air more
quickly.

To heat massage oil before and
while using, slip the plastic
bottle inside a heavy weight
plastic baggie and sit inside a jar
you have filled with very warm
water.

Soothe Aching Muscles
Peppermint 4 drops
Thyme 4 drops
Lavender 4 drops
Marjoram 3 drops
Carrier Oil 1 ounce

Blend the above essential oils in
a PET plastic bottle then add the
carrier oil or other carrier oils.
Massage lightly.

This blend can also be added
(about half) to the bath tub.
People with sensitive skin should
use cautiously as peppermint
can be a skin irritant.

Back Ache Massage
Lavender 10 drops
Rosemary 6 drops
Sandalwood 6 drops
Geranium 3 drops
Almond oil 1 ounce

Mix in an PET bottle, shake and
apply to areas of discomfort.
Massage in as desired

Sore Muscles?

Sweet Almond Oil 2 ounces
Black Pepper 12 drops
Marjoram 6 drops
Juniper berry 6 drops
Ginger 6 drops

Blend these oils together then use as a massage oil. You only need to use about a teaspoon or two for a nice massage.

Massage Oil For Sore Muscles

Allspice 5 drops
Cinnamon 4 drops
Cajeput 3 drops
Chamomile 3 drops
Carrier oil 1 tablespoon

Mix all oils, and use as you would any other massage oil.

Sore Muscles

Grapefruit 10 drops
Tea Tree 6 drops
Rose 5 drops
Spearmint 4 drops
Carrier oil 1 ounce

Mix together in a PET bottle and massage into sore muscles.

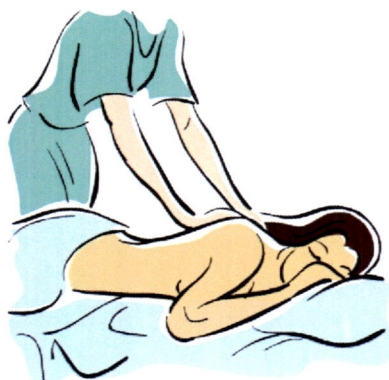

Sore Muscles #2

Black Pepper 12 drops
Marjoram 6 drops
Juniper berry 6 drops
Ginger 6 drops
Carrier oil 2 ounces

Blend these oils together and use as a massage oil. You only need to use a small amount.

Most people love the warming and penetrating heat these oils will produce.

If at anytime you feel this blend is too warming, then you should discontinue use or add more carrier oil before the next use.

Sore Muscles #3

Rosemary 10 drops
Peppermint 10 drops
Basil 5 drops
Sweet Almond 1 ounce

Mix together and add Sweet Almond oil. Shake well. Use this massage blend to work on sore muscles.

This recipe is especially good for sore back muscles.

Muscle Pain Help

Eucalyptus 10 drops
Peppermint 10 drops
Rosemary 10 drops
Ginger 10 drops
Black Pepper 10 drops
Sweet Almond Oil 2 ounce

Blend well in a PET bottle. Then massage area with just a little of the above blend.

Muscular Pain Rub
Cypress 15 drops
Juniper Berry 15 drops
Lavender 10 drops
Bay Laurel 5 drops
Rosemary 5 drops
Carrier Oil 2 ounces

Mix together in an glass bottle.
Then add to the carrier oil.
Massage a few drops as
needed on the sore muscles.

Muscle Soreness and Relaxing Massage Oil
Ylang-ylang 20 drops
Ginger 20 drops
Nutmeg 12 drops
Rosemary 8 drops
Sweet Almond Oil 2 ounces

Blend all essential oils together,
then add to the Sweet Almond
oil.

Warm oil slightly and massage
into sore muscles to help
relieve soreness by relaxation.

Sports Muscle Rub Blend
Lavender 5 drops
Peppermint 4 drops
Rosemary 6 drops
Helichrysum 4 drops
Apricot Kernel Oil 1 ounce

Blend all in a PET bottle, shake
well and rub into sore muscles.

Legs and feet-which will
normally take the brunt of
activities will love this blend.

For the Sport Enthusiast
Playing a little too much
badminton? Tennis? Or how
about all those water sport
activities?

In any case, you might get a few
sore muscles.

To help prevent injuries enjoy a
little rub down before you begin
your exercising with a few
essential oils blended into your
favorite carrier oil.

Muscle and Nerve Inflammation Massage
Lavender 8 drops
Roman Chamomile 4 drops
Helichrysum 4 drops
Marjoram 3 drops
Jojoba 2 ounces

Blend essential oils in a PET
plastic bottle. Once blended
then add the Jojoba or other
carrier oil of choice.

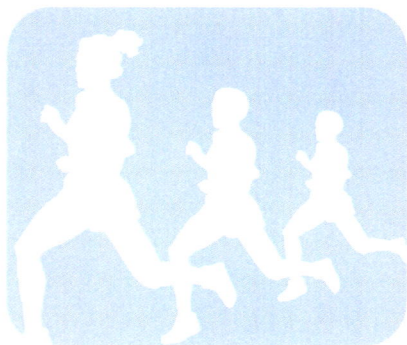

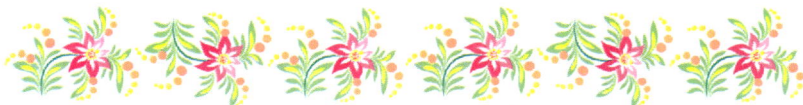

All Purpose Refreshing Disinfecting Blend

Lavender 20 drops
Peppermint 10 drops
Tea Tree 10 drops

Mix all oils together in an glass bottle. Add 8 drops to 1 ml of emulsifier. Shake well then add to 2 cups of distilled water.

Put all in a spray bottle.

You can use this spray to clean and disinfect the air.   Simply use as a room spray as needed. It is a light refreshing scent.

Kitchen Surface Sanitizer

Lemon 50 drops
Grapefruit 40 drops
Lime 40 drops
Tea Tree 20 drops
Emulsifier 2 teaspoons
Distilled Water 4 ounces

Place essential oils in a bottle, next add the emulsifier.

Blend well before adding the distilled water.

Use in a mist sprayer. Shake well before and during use.

Keep this blend handy for all your kitchen surfaces.

Take Along Travel Sanitizer

Lavender 30 drops
Clove bud 20 drops
Peppermint 15 drops
Patchouli 10 drops
Emulsifier 1 teaspoon
Distilled water 2 ounces

Blend the essential oils with the emulsifier and shake well. Add the 2 ounces of distilled water.

Shake well before spraying on any surface you wish to Sanitize. Such as toilet seats, bathtubs, sinks, door handles, and telephones. Leave on for 5-10 minutes then wipe off any residue.

Some essential oils when mixed with emulsifier may leave a slight film on the surface.

Room Disinfectant

Tea Tree 65 drops
Thyme 50 drops
Eucalyptus 35 drops
Emulsifier 2 teaspoons
Distilled Water 4 ounces

Mix essential oils with emulsifier then add the distilled water. Use a spray mister to spray the air.   Shake well and spray as often as desired.

HELPFUL HOUSEHOLD CLEANING TIP

Any of these blends of essential oils can also be added to your laundry. Blend just the essential oils, omit the emulsifier and distilled water. Then simply apply several drops to a small cloth and toss in your clothes dryer. If you prefer you can add several drops to the final rinse of your clothes washer too.

Forest Scented Room Disinfecting Freshener

Pine Needle 50 drops
Cinnamon 25 drops
Juniper berry 20 drops
Clove Bud 10 drops
Distilled water 4 ounces

Add the essential oils to the bottle of distilled water. Shake well, spray around room as necessary.

Mop Bucket Blend

Lemongrass 20 drops
Spruce 10 drops
Pine needle 10 drops
Cedarwood 5 drops
Patchouli 5 drops

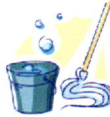

Blend these together then add to your mop bucket. This blend is great for getting rid of foul odors. When finished mopping, don't forget to let this run into your floor drain.

NOTES

Eliminate Odors In A Musty Basement Spray/Diffuser Blend

Spruce needle 50 drops
Eucalyptus 50 drops
Bay Rum 20 drops
Tea Tree 20 drops
Lime 10 drops
Lavender 10 drops
Cedarwood 10 drops
Emulsifier 10ml

Blend the above in an glass bottle, Pour into your spray bottle and add 4 ounces of water.

Shake well and spray onto any surface in your basement that appears to be growing the unwanted smell.

Spray some around the room too.

 As an alternative you can use just the essential oils (omit the emulsifier and water) this blend in any fan type diffuser.

Diffuse constantly for several days. Remember to keep adding more essential oils as they will be used up quickly in very smelly basements.

Mild Mildew Blend

Tea Tree Oil 2 teaspoons
Water 2 cups

Combine in a spray bottle, shake well to blend, and spray on problem areas. Do not rinse. Do not Spray on finished (painted or varnished) surfaces. It will destroy them.

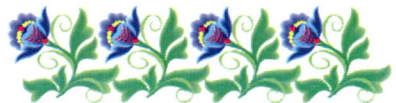

Mattress Sanitizer
Spearmint 50 drops
Thyme 15 drops
Cajeput 10 drops
Lemon 10 drops
Distilled Water 2 ounces

Shake and blend well. Spray on
mattresses and foundations.

Let dry thoroughly before
putting on the bedding,
approximately 1-2 hours.

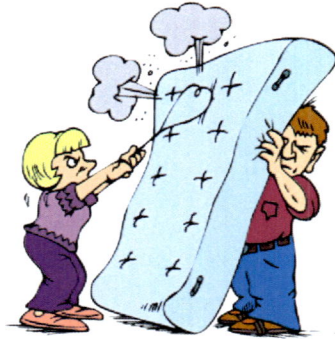

Mattress Spray
Peppermint 50 drops
Eucalyptus 10 drops
Oregano 10 drops
Pine 5 drops
Water 2 ounces

Shake well before and during
the spraying process. This will
make enough to spray the
mattress and foundation.

Your bedroom may smell very
strong, so you may want to
open a window after you are
finished or close the door and
let this blend sanitize the whole
room. Allow about 1-2 hours
drying time.

Bathroom Air Freshener
Peppermint 25 drops
Sandalwood 10 drops
Lavender 5 drops
Distilled Water 1 ounce

Add the above essential oils to a
spray top PET plastic bottle, add
the water.

Shake well. Spray in the
bathroom as desired.

Just So You Know!

Keep unused misting and
room spray in the refrigerator
for   future use.
Any room freshener can be
used to freshen the room
quickly and easily.
Discard any unused spray
after 30 days.. Or better yet,
just mix enough for a couple
weeks at a time.

Sick Room Disinfecting Spray
Bergamot 60 drops
Oregano 40 drops
Spearmint 25 drops
Cedarwood 15 drops
Cinnamon Leaf 10 drops
Emulsifier 5 mls
Distilled Water 4 ounces

Add essential oils and emulsifier
into a clean bottle and then
pour the distilled water into the
bottle.

Shake well then spray in the air.
Shake well before each use.

A Stimulating and Erotic Love Perfume

Jasmine Absolute 10 drops
Rose Absolute 10 drops
Ylang-Ylang 10 drops
Jojoba 1 ounce

Blend well, apply to pulse points.

A Light Romantic Perfume

Orange 8 drops
Cypress 5 drops
Juniper Berry 5 drops
Sandalwood 7 drops
Jojoba 1 tablespoon

Blend all the above oils in a glass perfume bottle. Let blend for a few days before using.

Romantic Hot Tub Blend

Ylang-Ylang Extra 10 drops
Sandalwood 10 drops
Rosewood 5 drops
Neroli 5 drops
Coconut Emulsifier 45 drops

Blend all together in a PET plastic bottle.   Then add 3-6 drops to your hot tub.

Since it is most likely you and your close friend. Start out with few drops of essential oils added to the tub.

Enjoy the moment– light a few candles too and play a little soft music.

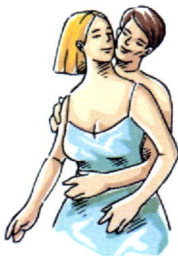

Romantic Massage #1

Cedarwood 2 drops
Clary sage 2 drops
Orange 1 drop
Vanilla 1 drop
Sunflower 1 ounce

Combine all these oils and shake well. Slowly massage into your partners skin. Take your time and massage out stressful areas, shoulders, back and more. Enjoy a quiet evening together.

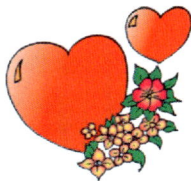

Romantic Massage #2

Jasmine 2 drops
Orange 2 drops
Sandalwood 2 drops
Ylang-ylang 1 drop
Almond Oil 1 ounce

Blend together and give a slow loving massage.

Loving Sweet Massage Oil

Sandalwood 12 drops
Ylang-ylang 6 drops
Clary Sage 4 drops
Rose 2 drops
Neroli 2 drops
Sweet Almond Oil 2 ounces

Blend all the essential oils and add to the warmed Sweet Almond oil. Apply to the body using comfortable pressures.

This blend **should not** be used on the genital area or on the face.

Massage For Mild Impotence

due to low Libido and Physical
Exhaustion
Ginger 2 drops
Cinnamon 1 drop
Coriander 1 drop
Rosemary 1 drop
Sunflower oil 1 tablespoon

Blend all together and massage
into the lower back, upper
abdominal area and upper
thighs. Avoid the genitals as
these oils can be very warm and
may irritate the sensitive skin in
this area.

Use this blend daily for 10 days
Also take a daily bath with
Ginger 2drops and Black Pepper
2 drops added to the water.

Romantic Massage Oil

Cedarwood 2 drops
Clary Sage 2 drops
Orange 1 drop
Vanilla 2 drops
Sunflower Oil 2 ounces

Combine all these oils and shake
well. Slowly massage into your
partners skin.

Take your time and massage out
stressful areas, shoulders, back
and more... Enjoy a quiet
evening together.

In The Mood For Love

Rose 2 drops
Sandalwood 3 drops
Massage Lotion 1-2 tablespoons

Apply on face, body, and arms
just prior to enjoying the
afternoon or evening together.

Light Sensual Lotion

Ylang-ylang 2 drops
Jasmine 2 drops
Bergamot FCF 2 drops
Unscented Lotion 1 tablespoon

Mix the above together and
enjoy your new one-of-a-kind
sensual lotion.

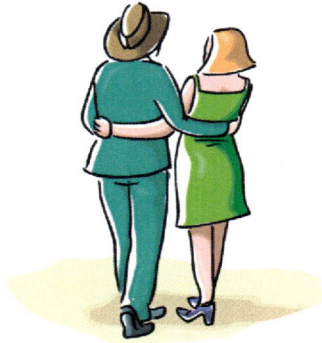

For a Romantic Massage

Ylang-ylang 10 drops
Sandalwood 5 drops
Black Pepper 3 drops
Ginger 2 drops
Sweet Almond oil 1 ounce

Mix all oils and add to the carrier
oil,. Shake well and warm gently
before massaging. Remember to
give a reciprocating massage.

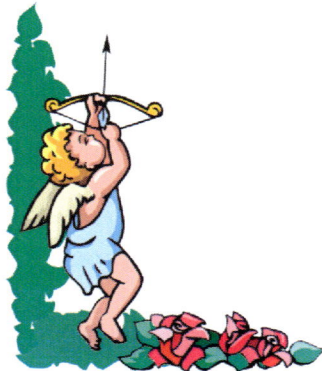

For A Romantic Dinner

Black Pepper 2 drops
Grapefruit 2 drops
Jasmine 2 drops

Use the above blend in your tea light diffuser, it will set the evenings atmosphere for what lies ahead!

Loving Massage For A Romantic Evening For Two

Cedarwood 5 drops
Jasmine 3 drops
Orange 3 drops
Ylang-Ylang 1 drop
Rose 1 drop
Sunflower oil 2 ounces

Blend together and enjoy as you give each other a loving massage.

Romantic Encounters For You

Ylang-ylang 8 drops
Jasmine 8 drops
Bergamot FCF 8 drops
Massage Lotion 2 ounces

Blend essential oils in an glass bottle. Then blend in the 2 ounces of massage lotion.

Simply enjoy as you give each other a massage.

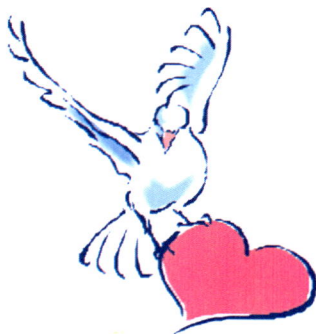

Sensuality Bath/Massage Blend

Rose 2 drops
Ylang-ylang 2 drops
Jasmine 1 drop
Neroli 1 drop
Clary Sage 2 drops
Sandalwood 2 drops

Fill the tub with warm water. Swirl water add the essential oils. Close the door for 5 minute and let the oils permeate the room.

Light a few candles, play some soft music. Enjoy a wonderful bath together.

You can mix the above essential oils in 1 ounce of carrier oil for a sensual massage.

The Sensual Bath

Sandalwood 3 drops
Rosewood 2 drops
Ylang-ylang 2 drops
Patchouli 1 drop
Neroli 1 drop

Fill the tub with warm water Swirl water and add the essential oils. Close the door for 5 minutes and let the oils permeate the room.
Light a few candles, play some soft music. Enjoy a wonderful bath together.

Sensuous Massage

Jasmine 5 drops
Mandarin 5 drops
Frankincense 5 drops
Sandalwood 5 drops
Apricot oil 2 ounces

Blend well and enjoy with a friend.

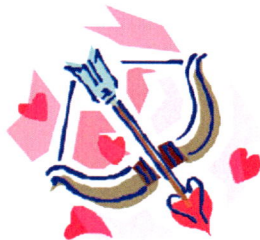

Romantic Air Freshener

Use in an aroma lamp with water.
Clary Sage 5 drops
Clove Bud 5 drops
Ylang-ylang 5 drops
Black Pepper 5 drops

Mix together, put in aroma lamp or blend up enough to use in you fan type diffuser.

Use about 5-10 drops of blend on a diffuser pad depending on the size of your rooms.

Aphrodisiac Bath

Jasmine 4 drops
Ginger 4 drops
Neroli 4 drops
Clary Sage 6 drops
Black Pepper 1 drop

Mix all essential oils then add half to a hot bath,

Use the rest the next time.

Or you can diffuse in the bedroom or other room of the house.

This blend can be used anytime but will be more fun with the one you love!

Romantic Massage Blend For A Hot August Night

Frankincense 12 drops
Ginger 4 drops
Coriander 3 drops
Ylang-ylang Extra 1 drop
Sweet Almond oil 2 ounces

Blend all ingredients.

This wonderful blend has inspired and stimulated many a romantic couple.

If the spark has weakened or slowed in your marriage– try using this blend as an after bath or massage blend to excite your partner.

Scents-ual Touch Massage Oil

Ginger 8 drops
Myrrh 5 drops
Jasmine 2 drops
Cardamom 1 drop
Carrier Oil 2 ounces

Mix all oils together and give one another a slow sensual massage. Please allow plenty of time!

Temptation Body Spray

Rose Absolute 6 drops
Neroli 6 drops
Jasmine Absolute 6 drops
Emulsifier 20 drops
Body Spray Base 2 ounces

To blend add the essential oils/ absolutes to an empty PET bottle then add the emulsifier, blend well. Then add 2 ounces of the body spray base.

Shake well before each use.

Carpet Cleaning and Deodorizer
Lavender 5 drops
Lemon 3 drops
Clary Sage 1 drop
Grapefruit 1 drop
Borax 6 Tablespoons

Mix all ingredients and sprinkle on carpet. Let sit for 5 – 10 minutes and vacuum thoroughly.

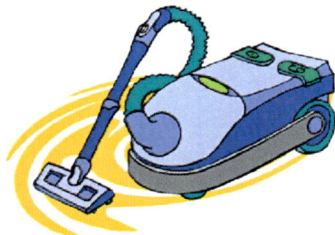

Carpet Deodorizing Freshener
Eucalyptus 30 drops
Cinnamon Leaf 30 drops
Lemon30 drops
Clove Bud 10 drops
Baking Soda 1 cup

Blend all oils and soda in a wide mouth jar and close the lid. Let set for 24 hours.

Sprinkle over carpet and let sit for 10-15 minutes.
Then vacuum.

Carpet Freshener
Orange 15 drops
Lavender 15 drops
Clove Bud 10 drop
Baking Soda 1 cup

Blend all the essential oils together and then mix into the baking soda. Seal tightly for 24 hours. Shake occasionally during this time period. Then sprinkle on your carpets. Let sit for 30 minutes, then vacuum.

Stinky Carpet Refresher
High humidity and all the bacteria and mold can lurk in your carpet can soon make the room smell badly. Mix this up and use before vacuuming to freshen not only the air but your carpet.

Lime 1 teaspoon
Tangerine 1/2 teaspoon
Ginger 1/4 teaspoon
Litsea Cubeba 1/4 teaspoon
Baking Soda 1 cup

Blend all the ingredient together in a glass pint jar.

Shake well, let blend for 24 hours. Then sprinkle on your carpet, let sit for 20-30 minute. Vacuum your carpet as usual.

HELPFUL HOUSEHOLD HINT
Store any remaining powder in a tightly covered jar in the refrigerator. You may need to make fresh if not used within 2-3 weeks.

Chest
Cinnamo
Rosemary
Pine 6 dr
Thyme 3

Blend the
use 4-5 d
water. In

Breat
Asth
Eucalypt
Pine Ne
Tea Tree
Frankinc
Myrrh 2
Thyme :
Jojoba

Global Crossing

Jan 25
Jun 15
das 5
Gift 5

e

Blend all oils in a 2 ounce PET plastic bottle. Rub on chest and mid-back as needed.

You can also mix just the essential oils (eliminate the jojoba) and inhale this blend from a personal inhaler or use in a diffuser.

For The Flu, Sinusitis, Bronchitis
Eucalyptus 30 drops
Lavender 15 drops
Pine 12 drops
Marjoram 6 drops
Thyme 3 drops

Mix all oils in an glass bottle. Then place 6 drops in a bowl of hot water and breath in the steam for 5-10 minutes.

Peppermint 5 drops
Thyme 5 drops
Sunflower oil 1 ounce

Mix well and gently rub on your chest and throat several times a day.

Another Bronchitis Blend
Thyme linalool 10 drops
Eucalyptus radiata 10 drops
Niaouli 10 drops
Myrtle 25 drops

Blend well and use in one of the following ways:

- Put about 5-10 drops in a bowl of steaming hot water and let the steam fill the air
- Or place several drops on a tissue or use in a personal inhaler,
- Or put 3-5 drops in a carrier oil and massage over the chest and back.

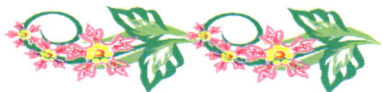

Bronchitis Foot Rub
Thyme 10 drops
Eucalyptus 10 drops
Cinnamon 2 drops
Nutmeg 2 drops
Ginger 2 drops
Sweet Almond 1 ounce

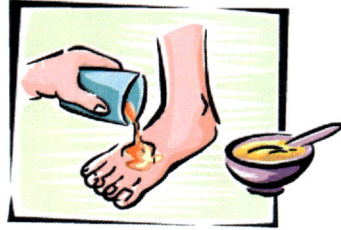

Blend all the essential oils together in a bottle, then add the almond oil. Rub a few drops of this mixture on the bottom of your feet twice a day.

Remember to wear socks to bed too. This may appear strange but remember essential oils are easily absorbed through the skin on the bottom of your feet.

The essential oils will quickly travel through the blood stream to the area they are needed to help. You get slow absorption all day and the essential oils will be working for you without having to constantly reapply.

Inhalation Formula
Eucalyptus 12 drops
Cedarwood 6 drops
Rosemary 3 drops
Peppermint 6 drops
Boiling water 2 cups

Pour blend into bottle, shake well and then add 5 drops to the boiling water. Place in a stainless steel bowl. Lean over the bowl and place a towel over head and inhale the oils.

Caution– Remember that sometimes more is not better when it comes to using essential oils especially with steam.

Cold Fighting Blend
Orange 15 drops
Eucalyptus 10 drops
Juniper Berry 10 drops
Pine Needle 10 drops
54, 6 drops
Rosewood 6 drops
Lemon 5 drops
Ginger 4 drops

Blend together and use in a diffuser or a few drops in a bath. Relax for 15-20 minutes. Then dry off well and wrap yourself in a thick robe, and go to bed early.

Cold Comfort
Eucalyptus radiata 10 drops
Eucalyptus globulus 5 drops
Ravensara 5 drops
Thyme 3 drops
Oregano 2 drops

Blend well then either place a few drops in a personal inhaler or diffuse into the air using any diffuser. Best if used every 3-4 hours.

Cold And Flu Bath
Lavender 3 drops
Bergamot FCF 3 drops
Tea Tree 2 drops
Eucalyptus 2 drops

Add the above essential oils to a hot bath.

Springtime Cold Relief

Eucalyptus 4 drops
Geranium 4 drops
Peppermint 4 drops
Rosemary 4 drops

Blend all ingredients in an glass bottle. This blend can then be used in a personal inhaler.

Or added to a bath– only about 4 drops. You can also add 5 drops to 1 ounce of carrier oil and rub on chest, neck, or other area you desire.

Just So You Know!

Remember all essential oils have antibacterial, antifungal, antimicrobial and antiseptic properties to varying degrees.

If there are odors caused from the growth of germs from any of these sources, the essential oils will help destroy the odor causing germs too.

Spray them Away!

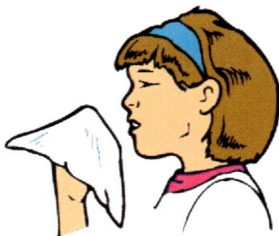

Sinus Steam Inhalation

Eucalyptus 2 drops
Tea Tree 2 drops
Ginger 1 drop
Thyme 1 drop
Steaming Water 1 quart

Pour hot water into a 2 quart bowl, add essential oils. Hold head over the bowl, drape a towel over head and bowl.

Breathe for 5-10 minutes. You may repeat this up to 6 times a day. You may not be able to breathe continually for the 5-10 minutes, so just take it slowly.

Breathe for a while then
 remove your head from "steam room" and then when ready after a minute return to "steam room."

Sore Throat Soothing Spray

Roman Chamomile 2 drops
Geranium 2 drops
Lemon 1 drop
Tea tree 1 drop
Pine 1 drop
1 tbsp. apple cider vinegar
1 tsp. honey
1/2 cup distilled water
(warmed)

Add the vinegar and the essential oils into the honey, then add to the warm water.

Stir well and add to a bottle with a spray nozzle. Spray 1-2 times into the back of the throat. It is okay to swallow.

But you should try not to eat or drink for at least 15 minutes after a spraying.

Spray as often as needed.

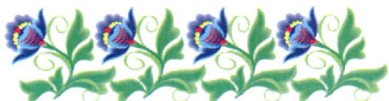

Summer Stuffiness With Cough

Myrtle 10 drops
Hyssop 3 drops
German Chamomile 3 drops

Blend well in an glass bottle and add to a personal inhaler or smell from the bottle. Do this several times a day.

If you are really stuffy and cant get any air through your nasal passages smell a little Peppermint a few minutes before smelling this blend.

The Peppermint will usually open up your nasal passage enough so you can inhale this blend.

Allergy Relief For Head Congestion

Eucalyptus 5 drops
Lavender 2 drops
Rosemary 2 drops
Peppermint 1 drop

Mix all essential oils together. Then add 1-3 drops to a personal inhaler or several drops in a fan or other room diffuser.

Hay Fever Help

Roman Chamomile 3 drops
German Chamomile 3 drops
Helichrysum 2 drops
Lavender 2 drops
Peppermint 1 drop (optional)

Blend together and put in a personal inhaler. Inhale once in each nostril about 6-8 hours during Hay fever Days!

Sinus Congestion (Due To Allergies)

Peppermint 5 drops
Roman Chamomile 5 drops
Rosemary 5 drops

Blend the above essential oils in an glass bottle. Then apply several drops inside a personal nasal inhaler.

Reassemble the inhaler and then place near your nostrils. Inhale a couple times in each nostril.

This will help to relieve the pressure, open the airways and the Chamomile may help to stop other allergy type reactions.

Just So You Know

It is strongly discourage to use tea light diffusers or candles when you are suffering with respiratory conditions as the small amount of soot produced by open flames can cause additional irritation to already irritated nose and throat.

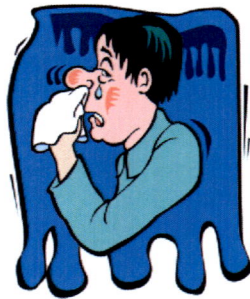

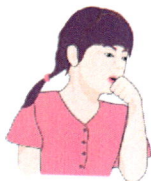

Dry Cough Blend
Eucalyptus globulus 8 drops
Myrtle 4 drops
Pine Needle 2 drops
Lemon 2 drops
Sweet Almond 1 ounce

Add to Sweet Almond Oil, rub on chest twice a day.

Flu and Cold Body Massage
Thyme linalool 5 drops
Ravensara 5 drops
Peppermint 5 drops
Naiouli 5 drops
Sweet Almond oil 1 oz

Blend well and massage the legs, arms, neck, chest, and back.

This is for adults and **children over 5** years. Dilute further with carrier oil if used on younger children.

 This is a fairly strong smelling massage blend. So please if you are using this, you should be staying at home in bed, not out in public.

Helpful Tip:
Use Eucalyptus (several drops) in a pan of water on low heat or put in vaporizer or diffuser. This will disperse into the room and help break up mucous and reduce coughing.

Open up your Sinuses Congestion Bath Blend
Eucalyptus 4 drops
Chamomile 4 drops
Anise 3 drops
Petitgrain 1 drop
Carrier oil of choice 5mls

Blend these oils together then while filling the bath tub use 5-6 drops of blend in the running water and enjoy!

Keep the bathroom door closed to keep the oils in the room.

Steam Room Blend
(For congestion)
Lavender 4 drops
Frankincense 2 drops
Eucalyptus radiata 2 drops

Blend together and place on a Terra Cotta Disc in the steam room.

Immune Boosting Massage Oil
Geranium 10 drops
Tea tree 10 drops
Lemon 8 drops
Thyme 8 drops
Myrrh 8 drops
Elemi 5 drops
Carrier oil 4 ounces

Blend essential oils together in a PET plastic bottle. Then add the carrier oil. Blend well.

Use to massage over body once or twice a day.

The essential oils in this blend will help your body to not only fight off unwelcome germs but will also help boost your immune system.

Insect Repellent!!

Geranium 10 drops
Cedarwood 5 drops
Bay laurel 5 drops
Lime 5 drops
Pine Needle 5 drops
Jojoba 2 ounces

Blend all oils well. Apply a few drops to palms of hands, then apply to area of exposed skin where the little pests may try to bite you.

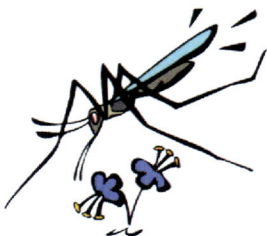

Insect Repellent #2

Bergamot FCF 4 drops
Pine needle 4 drops
Tea Tree 4 drops
Eucalyptus globulus 3 drops
Patchouli 2 drops
Peppermint 1 drop

Mix this blend and add to 1 ounce of sunflower oil of jojoba and apply on the skin before going out doors to repel insects (mainly mosquitoes) and keep them from bothering you.

If you will be in the sun, be sure to use Bergamot FCF as regular Bergamot can cause a terrible photosensitization reaction to occur in many people.

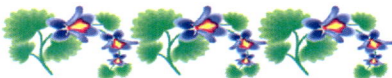

Insect Repellant #3

Eucalyptus Lemon 5 drops
Geranium 3 drops
Lavender 3 drops
Peppermint 1 drop
Sunflower Oil 1 tablespoon

Blend all in a PET plastic bottle. Apply as needed to exposed skin.

An alternative would be to mix the essential oils without adding the carrier oil.

Then apply one to two drops to the top of your shoes or bottom of your pant leg to deter the insects from biting you near you legs and feet.

Remember to flip the reeds over occasionally to refresh the scent.

Bug Repellent

Lemongrass 8 drops
Thyme 4 drops
Lavender 4 drops
Peppermint 4 drops

Blend all the essential oils in an glass bottle. This mixture can be placed (a couple drops) on a tissue and placed near your bedside or other area you wish to have bugs leave you alone.

You can also mix 4 drops per teaspoon of a light carrier oil and apply as a body rub,

OR add entire recipe to 1ml of emulsifier and once well blended add to 2 ounces distilled water and use as a spray.

Bug Off

Cajeput 25 drops
Lemon 19 drops
Geranium 19 drops
Cedarwood 13 drops
Sweet Almond Oil 2 ounces

Mix all the essential oils in a PET plastic bottle, then add the Almond oil. Shake well until blended. Apply a thin amount to exposed skin. Apply as needed.

Just So You Know!

Ticks are tough little bugs to repel. Especially since they crawl on the tips of their short legs.

We have had reports that Palmarosa works great when applied to your dogs collar.

Even dogs that spend a great deal of time outdoors. As for other blends, try Bug Off, applied to the dog's collar. (Recipe on above.)

Insect Repellant For Older Children And Adults

Eucalyptus 4 drops
Lavender 4 drops
Rosemary 4 drops
Tea Tree 4 drops
Fractionated Coconut 1 ounce

Blend well and apply as needed, around the face, neck, wrists, and anywhere those biting pests want to get you.

Because this blend is fairly strong and has many strong oils, **do not** use on children under 5 years or near or on infants.

Moth Away Blend

Cedarwood 30 drops
Sandalwood 30 drops
Lime 20 drops
Lavender 20 drops
Geranium 20 drops

Blend well and store in an glass bottle. Place several drops on your Terra Cotta Disc or Lavender sachet.

You may have to add more of this blend every 7-10 days depending on your infestation.

Patio Diffuser Oil #1
To Repel Insects

Lemongrass 5 ml
Citronella 3 ml
Geranium 2 ml

Patio Diffuser Blend #2
To Repel Insects

Lemongrass 5 ml
Thyme 2 ml
Lavender 2 ml
Peppermint 2 ml

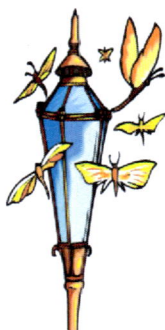

Blend either of the above recipes in a glass bottle.

Then place several drops in several tea light diffusers placed around your patio or porch.

Be sure to keep them full of water so the diffuser bowl won't burn dry and break.

Alternatively you can use and mix the above blends with unscented reed diffuser oil and place several reed diffusers around your patio and porch.

Soothe Insect Bites

Juniper 3 drops
Basil 2 drops
Lime 1 drop
Eucalyptus 1 drop
Sesame oil 1 teaspoon

Blend essential oils in carrier oil. Shake well and apply a small amount to the bites every few hours.

> ### JUST SO YOU KNOW
> If you continue to scratch a bug bite, histamines are being released, making it itch even more. You will eventually scratch yourself raw. Use cold compresses to help slow down the itch factor.

On The Bug Bite Blend

Roman Chamomile 5 drops
Eucalyptus 3 drops
Lavender 3 drops
Peppermint 2 drop
Apple Cider vinegar 1 ounce

Blend well, then add to
1 ounce cider vinegar.
Apply or dab on with a cotton ball to the insect bite area.

Can be used several times a day as needed.

Insect Bite Relief

Lavender 35 drops
Roman Chamomile 15 drops
Geranium 5 drops
Emulsifier 3 mls
Aloe Vera Liquid 2 ounces

Blend the essential oils with the emulsifier and then add to the Aloe Vera.

Apply to the area on and around the insect bite as needed every couple hours, using a cotton swab or cotton ball. Just dab on the bite area

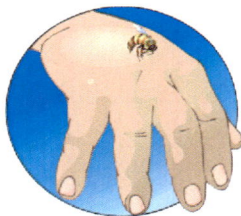

Alternative Bee Sting Oil

Roman Chamomile 5 drops
Lavender 5 drops
Fractionated Coconut oil -
1 teaspoon

Blend well in a small bottle and apply to the stung area 3 times a day or as needed.

> ### Helpful Tip:
> To keep bugs and other insects that crawl from entering your home. - Remember to spray a mixture of Peppermint essential oil and distilled water around windows and screens and on the threshold of your door entrances.
>
> Peppermint will also deter those little furry mice and moles from entering the home. The biggest inconvenience is it must be applied frequently to be effective.

Bug Infested Plant Spray #1

Sage 45 drops
Thyme 45 drops
Emulsifier 5 ml
Distilled Water 4 ounces

Mix essential oils with the emulsifier then add to the distilled water. Shake well and spray on your infected plants.

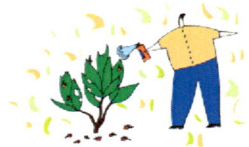

Bug Infested Plant Spray #2

Lavender 50 drops
Fennel 40 drops
Emulsifier 5 ml
Distilled Water 4 ounces

Mix essential oils with the emulsifier then add to the distilled water. Shake well and spray on your infected plants.

Please be sure to keep all Plant Sprays refrigerated between uses and try to use within 2 weeks or mix fresh

Anti-Fungal Spray For the Yard and Garden

Tea Tree 10 drops
Cinnamon 10 drops
Niaouli 10 drops
Water 1 gallon

Shake well and spray on surfaces (outdoor) that have been cleaned and dried where mold and mildew was present.

Allow this blend to dry without rinsing.

Garden Plant Spray For Those Pesky Bugs

Lemongrass 40 drops
Lavender 40 drops
Rosemary 10 drops
Geranium 10 drops
Emulsifier 1 tablepoon
Distilled Water 4 ounces

Blend the essential oils and emulsifier together, next add the distilled water. Shake well.

This spray is to be used on outdoor or house plants that have been or might become infested by little bugs. You do not need to soak the plant. Just a few mists should take care of them. Repeat every 2-3 days, or as needed.

Do not spray or use on the skin, as this is too concentrated for use on people or animals.

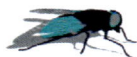

Household Fly Spray

Eucalyptus 40 drops
Lemon 20 drops
Peppermint 20 drops
Emulsifier 1/2 teaspoon
Linen Spray 4 ounces
PET bottle with spray top

Blend essential oils in PET plastic bottle, then add 1/2 teaspoon emulsifier. Mix thoroughly. Then add the linen spray and shake well. Spray around the room.

Before spraying on fabrics do a test spray to make sure the fabric and colors are not

Flea Bath For Your Dog
Tea Tree 6 drops
Pennyroyal 4 drops
Mild shampoo 2 ounces

Blend essential oils into the shampoo. Then Shampoo your dog OUTDOORS, lathering them well.

Any fleas, will try to 'flea' the dog when you give him the bath and you probably don't want any more fleas in the house.

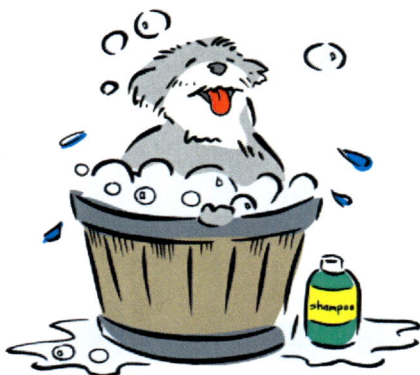

Rinse your pet well and completely dry the fur.

You can give this bath no more than once a week.

Do not use this on your cat!! Cats can't process essential oils through their liver and using essential oils directly on a cat could make the animal seriously ill.

Flea Oil Blend For Dogs
Peppermint 7 drops
Clary Sage 4 drops
Lemon 3 drops
Citronella 1 drop
Sweet Almond 1 tablespoon

Mix well and apply several drops to the neck, chest, legs and base of the tail of your dog.

You can also apply this blend to a bandanna or a cotton collar.

Pet Odors
Orange 10 drops
Lavender 10 drops
Tea Tree 6 drops
Lemon 5 drops
Geranium 5 drops
Nutmeg 2 drops
Neroli 3 drops

Blend these oils together, then use 4-5 drops in any diffuser.

Helpful Tip:

A Geranium plant in the house helps to repel insects and bugs.

NOTES

Keep The Pests Away Idea!

Cedarwood 3 ml
Pennyroyal 3 ml
Peppermint 3 ml
Lavender Sachets (several)

Blend the essential oils together in an glass bottle.

Take the Lavender Sachets and place them in a glass jar after applying several drops (5-8) of the above blend on the outside covering.

Keep tightly sealed for at least 24 hours.

Then strategically place the Sachets anywhere you know 'pests' such as mice and other insects like to enter your home.

Reapply to the Sachets every 2-3 weeks as needed, and simply follow the above steps.

Garden Pest
All Purpose Spray

Peppermint 25 drops
Rosemary 25 drops
Geranium 25 drops
Water 1 cup
Dish soap 1/2 teaspoon

Mix the essential oils and soap, stir well. Put this solution in your garden sprayer and head out to the garden.

Spray plants that appear to be infested with pests or as a general all purpose spray to avoid problems.

Keep any left over spray in a cool place, (refrigerate if possible). Use within 2 weeks or mix fresh each time.

NOTES

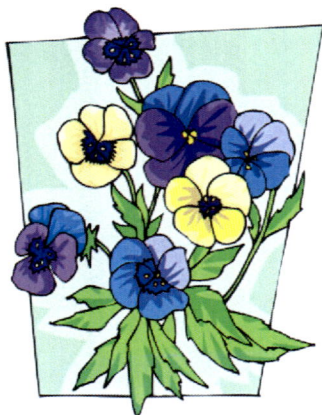

Breath Freshening Mouthwash

Myrrh 1 drops
Tea Tree 1drop
Peppermint 1drop
Distilled Water 2 ounces

Mix together in a plastic PET bottle. Shake well, then swish about 1 ounce in your mouth after brushing your teeth or after eating as needed.
Shake well before using.

Simple Refreshing Mouth Wash

Lemon 4 drops
Peppermint 2 drops

Add to 1 cup distilled water, shake well before each use. Swish a mouthful for about 1 minute and spit out.

This is an interestingly refreshing mouth rinse.

Therapeutic Gum Mouthwash

Myrrh 6 drops
Tea Tree 10 drops
Peppermint 1 drop
Lemon 3 drops
Grapeseed oil 1 teaspoon

Mix together and apply a small amount on your gums once a day, after brushing your teeth and rinsing your mouth with one of the above mouth-washes.

If the irritation, or gums do not heal, please see your dentist as you may have a very serious oral health issue.

Mouth Injury Blend

Peppermint 3 drops
Bergamot 3 drops
Tea Tree 1 drop
Myrrh 1 drop

Blend these essential oils together, then add 2 drops to 1 ounce of water that you have added 1 teaspoon of natural (raw) honey. Stir well.

Then swish and hold in your mouth for about one minute before spitting out.

Repeat 3 times a day, preferably after eating.

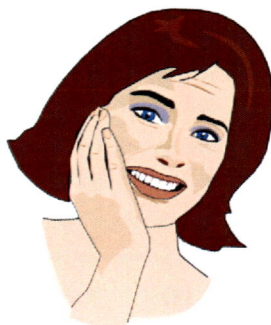

Toothache Oil

Tea Tree 6 drops
Chamomile 4 drops
Myrrh 2 drops
Peppermint 2 drops
Carrier oil 1 tablespoon

Place all oils in a clean container, shake to blend.

Apply on aching tooth and surrounding gum.

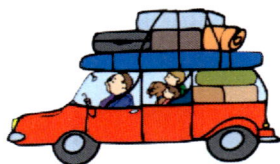

Motion Sickness Blend #1
Nutmeg 4 drops
Ginger 3 drops
Tangerine 6 drops
Roman Chamomile 3 drops
Cardamom 2 drops

Blend together. Place 1-2 drops on a cotton ball and inhale several whiffs prior to and while traveling.

Motion Sickness Blend #2
Roman Chamomile 10 drops
Ginger 10 drops
Peppermint 10 drops
Fennel 3 drops

Blend all essential oils in an glass bottle. Simply breathe a few drops from a tissue or use a personal inhaler.

Inhale 20-30 minutes before departure and also every few minutes while traveling.

Motion Sickness #3
Basil 1 drop
Peppermint 1 drop
Lavender 1 drop
Carrier Oil 2 teaspoons

Mix the oils together in the carrier oil, then rub your hands together to warm the oil.

Gently massage over the abdomen, afterwards you may want to cup your hands over your nose and mouth and slowly inhale for a few breaths before washing your hands.

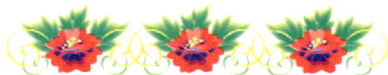

Appetite Suppressing Tummy Rub
Fennel 10 drops
Bergamot FCF 5 drops
Dill seed 5 drops
Patchouli 3 drops
Sunflower oil 1 tablespoon

Place all in a bottle and mix well. Massage a small amount of this blend on your stomach and abdominal area and massage lightly in a clockwise direction.

You can do this several times a day.

Quiet Down The Holiday Excited Kids Blend

Mandarin 20 drops
Marjoram 15 drops
Lavender 15 drop
Cedarwood 10 drops
Roman Chamomile 10 drops

Blend all in an glass bottle. Then diffuse a few drops about an hour before bedtime.

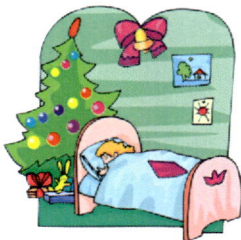

Christmas Mediation

Frankincense 5 drops
Myrrh 5 drops
Orange 5 drops

Mix all together and diffuse while just sitting and enjoying the season.

Helpful Tip

Family traditions are things families do every year on the same Holiday.

When you fix the same food for that special occasion year after year, baking desserts and decorating the home. Start a new Family tradition and diffuse the same essential oil blends year after year.

The "Lock and Key" mechanism of the brain will trigger fond memories many years from now.

Sweet Holidays

Cedarwood 4 drops
Fennel 2 drops
Lemon 2 drops
Orange 2 drops
Vanilla 2 drops

Mix all together. This blend works well in any diffuser, or mix with distilled water and use as a room spray.

Christmas Eve blend

Cedarwood 5 drops
Chamomile 3 drops
Geranium 3 drops
Orange 3 drops
Lavender 3 drops

Place in any diffuser and enjoy. This is a very peaceful blend and will help to relax you and the children for a Long winter's Sleep! Well, at least until Christmas morning!

Christmas Spritzer

Fir Needle 4 drops
Orange 2 drops
Cinnamon 1 drop
Distilled Water 1 cup

Blend well in a spray bottle. Shake well before using. Spray around the house as needed.

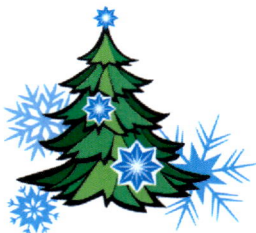

Season's Greetings Blend

Pine 8 drops
Lavender 3 drops
Sandalwood 3 drops
Frankincense 2 drops
Nutmeg 1 drop
Mandarin 1 drop

Blend all oils in an glass bottle and use in diffuser or place 5-6 drops on a cotton ball or add to you r potpourri.

Holiday Carpet Scent

Pine 15 drops
Spruce 10 drops
Spearmint 5 drops
Peppermint 2 drops

Blend all the above essential oils, then add all to a Scentball pad. Take this pad and add to a jar with 1/2 cup baking soda in it. Shake well and let sit for a few hours. Then sprinkle on the carpet. Let sit for 1/2 hour if possible. Then vacuum.

This is a clean refreshing scent and you may want to just put it in a diffuser to enjoy it that way too.

Sweet Holiday Dreams

Cedarwood 10 drops
Roman Chamomile 5 drops
Geranium 5 drops
Mandarin 5 drops

Mix well and add a drop to each pillow about 30 minutes prior to retiring for the night.

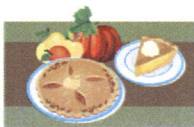

Holiday Mist Sprays

Clove Bud 40 drops
Cinnamon 30 drops
Ginger 30 drops
Orange 20 drops
Emulsifier 2 teaspoons

Blend essential oils with emulsifier.
Mix with 4 ounces of pure distilled water, shake well and mist.

Holiday Candy Scent

Peppermint 5 drops
Grapefruit 5 drops
Cinnamon 2 drops
Anise 1 drop

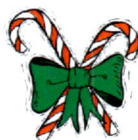

Blend this mix then diffuse. It's great!

Festive Blend

Spruce Needle 25 drops
Peppermint 20 drops
Anise 6 drops

Mix all oils together in a glass bottle. Use 3-4 drops in any diffuser as desired.

Festive Blend 2

Peppermint 35 drops
Frankincense 10 drops
Rosemary 5 drops

Mix all oils together in an glass bottle. Use 3-4 drops in any diffuser as desired

Simple Holiday Potpourri

Orange 10 drops
Clove bud 2 drops
Cinnamon 2 drops

Blend well and add a few drops to a diffuser or simmering pot.

Meditation Blend #1

Frankincense 10 drops
Sandalwood 6 drops
Clary Sage 6 drops
Myrrh 4 drops
Clove Bud 2 drops
Cistus 2 drops
Rose Otto 2 drops

Blend oils in an glass bottle, shake well. Add 2-6 drops to your diffuser for use while meditating.

The oils in this blend are very soothing and relaxing.

If you have a large room, you may need to use more oils in the diffuser.

Meditation Blend #2

Neroli 10 drops
Lemon 10 drops
Sandalwood 5 drops
Ylang-ylang 3 drops
Frankincense 3 drops
Myrrh 1 drop

Blend all together in an glass bottle. Then diffuse 5 drops in the room you are sitting in.

Add more oils if needed depending on the size of your room. Breath deeply, relax and enjoy while you meditate or just sit and relax.

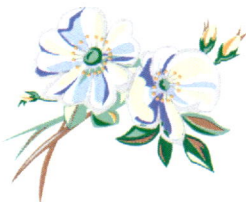

Meditation Blend #3

Lemon 15 drops
Lavender 5 drops
Juniper 5 drops
Geranium 5 drops
Frankincense 3 drops

Blend together, diffuse using any diffuser. It best to start with only 5-6 drops, more can always be added to your diffuser.

Relaxation Blend #1

Lemon 4 drops
Clary Sage 2 drops
Vetiver 1 drop

Simply add these drops to your diffuser and enjoy for the evening (or whenever you want to relax.)

Relaxation Blend #2

Mandarin 8 drops
Neroli 3 drops
Ylang-ylang 3 drops

Blend well and diffuse.

Relaxation Blend #3

Bergamot 10 drops
Rose Otto 2 drops
Roman Chamomile 3 drops

Blend well and diffuse

The above three recipes can be added to 2 ounces of distilled water, shake well and use in a spray bottle for a room freshener.

Or add to a warm tub of water for a nice relaxing bath.

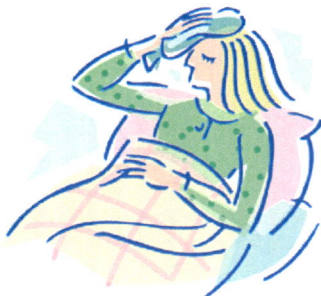

Headache Oil

Lavender 10 drops
Peppermint 5 drops
Sweet Almond oil 1 tablespoon

Blend well and massage on the temples, back of neck, and shoulder areas.

Headache Remedy!!

Marjoram 15 drops
Thyme 15 drops
Rosemary 15 drops
Peppermint 15 drops
Lavender 15 drops

Combine essential oils in a glass bottle. Depending on the strength desired, add 4-9 drops into any diffuser.

Lay quiet and relax.

Helpful Tip
Dehydration can cause headaches too.
Did you drink a full glass of plain water recently?

Try drinking some cool fresh water. Something as simple as that along with other remedies can make you feel better sooner.
You'll be surprised at what water can do!

Happiness and Joy #1

Geranium 10 drops
Ginger 10 drops
Tangerine 5 drops
Cinnamon 5 drops

Blend and diffuse in any room.

Happiness and Joy #2

Mandarin 15 drops
Orange 10 drops
Rose 5 drops
Jasmine 5 drops
Clove Bud 1 drop

Blend well, diffuse in any room or put 5-6 drops in a warm bath. Enjoy!

NOTES

Menstrual Cramp Relief
Clary Sage 9 drops
Fennel 5 drops
Geranium 3 drops
Peppermint 1 drop
Sunflower oil 1 ounce

Mix all oils together in a PET plastic bottle. Then rub gently on your abdomen as needed.

For Women Only
Lavender 10 drops
Mandarin 6 drops
Marjoram 5 drops
Cypress 4 drops
Sweet Almond 1 ounce
Jojoba 1 ounce

This blend is used to help ease night sweats and promote sleep. In an glass bottle, add the essential oils and carrier oils and shake well.

Apply nightly on chest and neck areas. This is a body oil and can be used freely on the body

.A Nice Bath For PMS
Lavender 5 drops
Geranium 2 drops
Grapefruit 2 drops
Clary Sage 1 drop
Epsom Salts 1-2 cups

Add the Epsom salts to the bath tub while it fills. Then add the essential oils. Swish around in the water. Then close the door and relax and enjoy your bath.

The Epsom salts should help with fluid retention and any muscles that may be cramping.

Uplifting Blend For Women
Bergamot 3 drops
Myrrh 2 drops
Ylang-ylang 2 drops
Fennel 4 drops
Geranium 4 drops

Blend all essential oils in a glass bottle Mix well the diffuse or use in your bath. Just enjoy!

PMS Bath Please Don't Disturb!
Lavender 15 drops
Geranium 9 drops
Grapefruit 9 drops
Clary sage 6 drops
Rose Otto 2 drops

Mix all oils in an glass bottle. Use 10 drops in your bath water. Be sure to add 1-2 cups Epsom salts to the water while tub is filling.

Epsom salts help to reduce swelling, bloating, and other aches and pains.
Soak for 20-30 minutes if possible. Undisturbed!!

Keep the door closed to the bathroom to help the oils stay in the room. Make the water as hot or as warm as you desire.

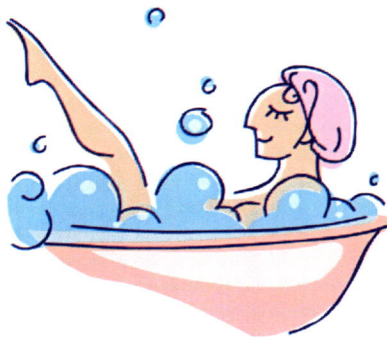

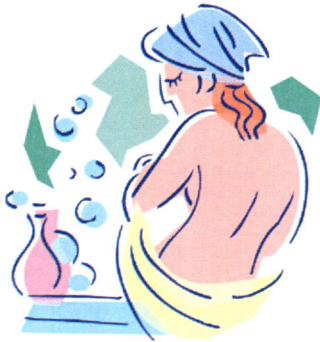

Premenstrual Syndrome Blend
Roman Chamomile 7 drops
Geranium 7 drops
Lavender 7 drops
Clary Sage 4 drops
Rose Otto 2 drops
Jojoba 1 ounce

Blend together and use a few days before the onset of your period, massage into lower back at least once a day.

For PMS And Depression
Clary Sage 12 drops
Rose 9 drops
Bergamot 9 drops
Neroli 6 drops

Blend together and add 3-4 drops in bath daily. You may also want to add a carrier oil to your bath water.

Balance and Relaxing Bath Blend
Geranium 4 drops
Lavender 4 drops
Cedarwood 1 drop
Vetiver 1 drop

Add to a warm bathtub, soak for 20 –30 minutes.
Enjoy and Relax!

Simple Morning Sickness Help
Add 4-6 drops of Spearmint to a terra cotta or other passive style diffuser near your bed.

Spearmint is milder to use than Peppermint and often times will ease a queasy stomach.

Pregnancy Back Ache Rub
Lavender 5 drops
Rosemary 3 drops
Sandalwood 3 drops
Geranium 1 drop
Sweet Almond Oil 2 ounces

Mix all essential oils in a bottle, then add the Sweet almond oil. Blend well.

Use to massage the lower back especially as needed during labor.

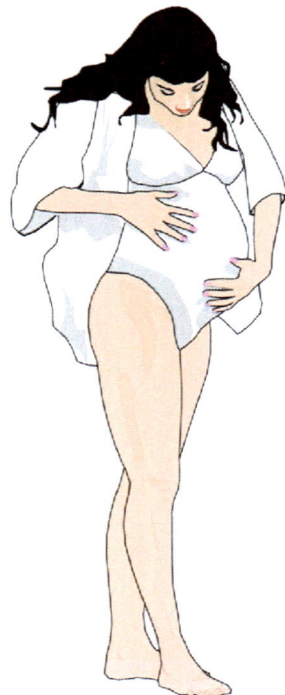

Instead Of All Those Cups Of Coffee

Black Spruce 5 mls
Cedarwood 2 mls
Peppermint 1 ml
Shower gel,
lotion or carrier
oil 4 ounces

Blend well in
your choice of
base product.
Use first thing in
the morning as you shower, this
will be invigorating when
blended in your shower gel.

If you prefer you can add to a
lotion or other carrier oil (use
only 1/2 the amount of the
essential oils if used in the lotion
or carrier oil) and apply a small
amount all over your body.

Suggestion: Mix a small amount
of this blend before mixing up a
large batch, just to make sure
you like it.

Wake Me Up Blend

Orange 3 drops
Clary Sage 2 drops
Coriander 2 drops
Helichrysum 1 drop
Jasmine Absolute 1 drop
Palmarosa 1 drop
Vetiver 1 drop
Jojoba 1 teaspoon

Blend all together and wear as
a perfume. Inhale as needed.

Can also be used on a Terra
Cotta pendant or in other
aromatherapy jewelry but omit
the Jojoba if you use on jewelry.

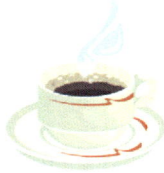

A Little Uplifter

Clary Sage 4 drops
Ylang-ylang 4 drops
Geranium 3 drops
Basil 2 drops
Sandalwood 1 drop

Mix in an glass bottle and use in
an atomizer or diffuser. Or if
desired place 4-6 drops in an
aroma lamp.

Here's A Good "Pick Me Up"

(If you are feeling down)
Lavender 8 drops
Ylang-ylang 8 drops
Basil 2 drops
Geranium 2 drops
Bergamot 2 drops
Jojoba 1 ounce

Mix the above ingredients in a
small glass bottle. Then apply a
small amount on back of hands
and pressure points on front of
hands. Use 2-3 times daily.

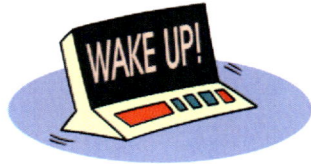

Stimulating Morning Blend

Rosemary 3 drops
Basil 2 drops
Juniper 1 drop
Peppermint 1 drop

Blend all in a small bottle. Then
add to your morning bath or
apply to your shower sponge
and rub vigorously over your
entire body. Enjoying the
wonderful smell these oils
provide.

Alertness Mist Spray

Bergamot 40 drops
Grapefruit 40 drops
Peppermint 40 drops
Juniper Berry 30 drops
Lavender 25 drops
Emulsifier 2 teaspoons
Pure Water 4 ounces

Shake and spray from a mist sprayer.

Alertness Massage

Ginger 6 drops
Grapefruit 5 drops
Juniper Berry 4 drops
Carrier Oil 15 mls

Blend together. Shake well and use as needed.

Office Blend-Afternoon Pick Me Up!

1-2 drops each of Lavender and Grapefruit placed in your desktop diffuser or on a cotton ball or in a personal inhaler.

Although diffusing it in the entire office will keep everyone busy working instead of sleeping.

To Help With Depression

Rose 10 drops
Neroli 2 drops
Sandalwood 3 drops
Almond Oil 1 ounce

Mix all together in an empty bottle. Then apply a small amount on hands, arms or legs and massage in. This blend can be used as often as needed.

In Times Of Grief

Neroli 4 drops
Roman Chamomile 2 drops
Jasmine 2 drops
Rose 1 drop
Jojoba oil 4 mls

Blend all the above oils together.

Can be worn as a fragrance-like perfume or inhale from the bottle.

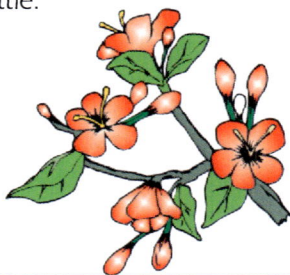

NOTES

Antiseptic Cream

Lavender 40 drops
Tea Tree 20 drops
Roman Chamomile 10 drops
Lemon 10 drops
Sorbolene Cream 2 ounces

Blend the essential oils
together in an glass bottle.
Then mix all these with the
2 ounces of sorbolene cream.

Apply a small amount to cuts
and abrasions as needed. May
be covered up with a band aid
if needed.

Cracked Skin Soak

Tea Tree 4 drops
Myrrh 2 drops
Lavender 4 drops

Mix these oils in 2 ounces of
Hazelnut oil. Then warm this
blend slightly.

Apply this warm mixture to
your hand. If you can, place in
a small bowl, just large enough
to fit your hands.

Continue to smooth on this
mixture and soak your hands
in this for up to 20 minutes.

Wipe off the excess (do not
wash your hands-just wipe off)
and put on your cotton gloves.

Leaving on overnight. Do this
for several nights .

You can reuse the oil mixture if
you want or make up new
each night.

First Aid Skin Wash And/Or Cream

Geranium 6 drops
Lavender 6 drops
Roman Chamomile 4 drops
Lemon 4 drops
Tea Tree 2 drops
Basin of warm water
Or add to Sorbolene Cream 2 oz

Blend together then store in a
cool place. Add several drops to a
basin of tepid water. Use this to
cleanse the wound area.

Alternately, you can add this
blend to one ounce of sorbolene
cream, blend well and then you
can apply a light coating of this
several times a day if needed to
the wound.

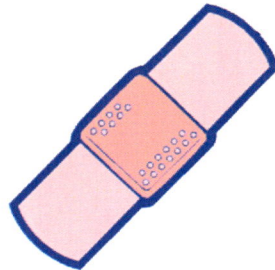

Antiseptic Wound Wash

Elemi 20 drops
Rosemary 10 drops
Lavender 10 drops
Myrrh 5 drops

Blend oils and add 20 drops to 2
cups of cooled, boiled water.
Bathe cuts (wounds) 3 times daily
with a sterile gauze.

Simple First Aid Wash

Simply put several drops of Lavender essential oil in a small basin of tepid water.

If the body part that needs cleaning is easy to submerse, simply swish around in the water for a few minutes.

If the body part cannot be submersed, then use a wash cloth and gently wipe over the area.

The natural antiseptic properties of Lavender will help fight any infection and its analgesic property will help with any pain or discomfort.

Use this wash for scrapes, bug bites, and any other bump or bruise.

Bacterial Skin Irritations

Geranium 5 drops
Lavender 4 drops
Bergamot FCF 3 drops
Sweet Almond oil or
Sunflower oil 1 ounce

Clean and dry the affected areas well, apply a blend of the above mixture.

Apply morning and night until healed. If no improvement after a day or two, you may need to seek medical attention.

Diaper Rash Powder

Lavender 5 drops
Cornstarch 2 tablespoons

Place the Lavender on a small piece of cloth or cotton ball and place in a small jar of cornstarch. Shake well and let blend for 24 hours.

Use this as needed at each diaper change. Do not shake this on. Use a small cloth or tissue to lightly rub on the diaper area.

Diaper Rash Oil

Lavender 10 drops
Roman Chamomile 1 drop
Sweet Almond 2 ounces

Blend well and apply a light amount on the babies' bottom.

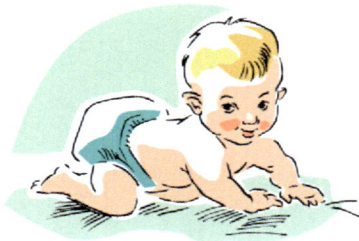

Diaper Rash Cream

Lavender 9 drops
Roman Chamomile 6 drops
Tea Tree 2 drops
Rose Otto 1 drop
Sorbolene Cream 4 ounces
Apricot oil 1 1/2 ounces

Blend the above ingredients together well and use a small amount between each diaper change or after bath time.

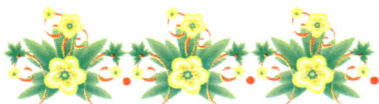

Bruise Blend

Geranium 4 drops
Helichrysum 2 drops
Juniper Berry 2 drops
Lavender 2 drops
Ginger 1 drop
Carrier oil 1 ounce

Mix all in a bottle and gentle mix together. Apply to bruised area several times a day.

Pain Relief For Bruises and To Help Reduce Swelling

Lavender 15 drops
Juniper Berry 10 drops
Marjoram 10 drops
Helichrysum 5 drops

Blend essential oils in an glass bottle. Place several drops in a cool basin of water and using a soft cloth apply the compress to the painful area for 15-20 minutes. Repeat every few hours as needed. OR

Mix the above essential oils in 2 ounces of fractionated coconut oil and apply several drops to the bruised area.

Apply using light pressure only– As you do not want to cause further tissue damage.

For General Bruising

Hyssop 10 drops
Cypress 10 drops
Geranium 8 drops
Lavender 2 drops
Sweet Almond or Sunflower oil 1 ounce

Blend well and apply to bruised areas several times a day.

Scars Blend

Helichrysum 10 drops
Sage 10 drops
Rosehip Seed Oil 1 ounce
Hazelnut Oil 1 ounce

Mix together. Apply at least 2 times daily to the scar.

This blend should help your wound heal with minimal scarring in about ten days.

Scar Lightening Blend

Helichrysum 1 ml
Lavender 1 ml
Sage 10 drops
Neroli 5 drops
Rosehip seed oil 1 ounce
Hazelnut oil 1 ounce

Mix until well blended, apply to the scar 2-3 times a day or until your scar has lightened and healed.

This blend is great to use on surgical scars. It will lighten and heal them quickly—but do not use until the sutures are out!

Bruise Diminishing Blend

Helichrysum 10 drops
Lavender 5 drops
Marjoram 4 drops
Geranium 3 drops
Juniper 2 drops
Thyme 2 drops
Jojoba 2 ounces

Blend well and apply to the bruised area several times a day.

Try to keep from bumping this area to prevent further tissue damage.

Dandruff Blend

Cedarwood 3 drops
Rosemary 3 drops
Tea Tree 3 drops
Olive oil 2 tablespoons

Blend all together. Then massage this into the scalp and hair. Be sure you reach all your scalp and your hair down to the ends. Wrap your head in a towel, and relax for about an hour. Then Shampooing using a mild shampoo.

Next rinse your hair using this recipe.

Distilled Water 1 cup
Cider Vinegar 1 tablespoon
Cedarwood 5 drops
Rosemary 10 drops

Mix well by vigorously shaking, then use to rinse your hair after shampooing. You do not need to rinse this rinse out. The smell of vinegar will dissipate once your hair is dry.

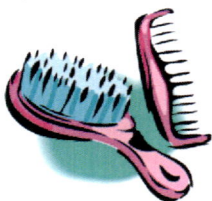

Dandruff Blend #2

Tea Tree 10 drops
Rosemary 8 drops
Cedarwood 6 drops
Pine Needle 4 drops
Basil 2 drops
Jojoba 2 ounces

Blend all together in a PET bottle. Massage some of this blend into your clean scalp and leave it on for at least thirty minutes or overnight. Then shampoo with a mild unscented shampoo.

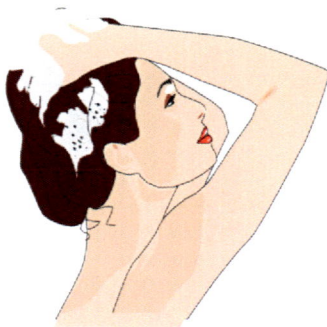

Dandruff Fewer Flakes Shampoo

Tea Tree 30 drops
Cedarwood 25 drops
Pine Needle 20 drops
Rosemary 20 drops
Clary Sage 20 drops
Lemon 20 drops
Unscented shampoo 8 ounces

Add the essential oils to the unscented shampoo and blend well.

Use this to shampoo your hair and scalp daily.

Just So You Know!

Most useful essential oils for dandruff include Rosemary, Bay Laurel, Lavender, Basil, Carrotseed, Cedarwood, Clary Sage, Cypress, Eucalyptus, Lemon, Patchouli, Sage and Tea Tree.

For Oily Hair
Ylang-ylang 9 drops
Lime 9 drops
Rosemary 8 drops
Grape seed Oil 2 tablespoons

Mix all ingredients then apply one teaspoon to hair and scalp and massage in.

Allow to penetrate for several hours or overnight. Wash your hair with a natural unscented shampoo washing it twice. Use three times a week.

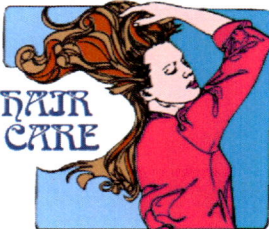

Hair Tonic
Basil 20 drops
Cedarwood 10 drops
Rosemary 10 drops
Jojoba 1 ounce

Blend oils together, massage a 1 teaspoonful into scalp nightly.

It will not leave the hair feeling greasy. Shampoo as normal in the morning

Sweet Smelling Hair
Rosewood 10 drops
Cedarwood 10 drops
Rosemary 10 drops
Conditioner 4 ounces

Blend all well. Apply to your hair after shampooing. Leave on for 3-5 minutes. Rinse thoroughly.

Scalp Massage
Lavender 10 drops
Clary Sage 6 drops
Rosemary 6 drops
Jojoba 1 tablespoon

Blend all ingredients in an glass bottle. Gently warm the bottle in a basin of warm water.

Apply a few drops to scalp, massage gently. Let absorb, then shampoo and style as you normally would.

Dry Or Damaged Hair
Clary Sage 3 drops
Cedarwood 1 drop
Rosemary 3 drops
Geranium 1 drop
Lavender 1 drop
Jojoba 1 tablespoon
Almond Oil 1 tablespoon

Mix oils in with carrier oils. Massage the blend into dry hair and scalp. Wrap head in towel and relax for an hour.

Shampoo with mild or unscented shampoo and then rinse well.

Alternative method is to add a few drops of the above oils to your shampoo and use on a regular basis.

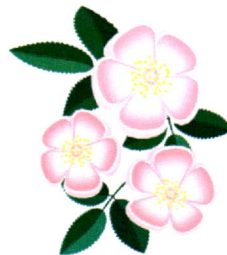

Fatigue Relief Massage Blend

Peppermint 6 drops
Rosemary 5 drops
Grapefruit 4 drops
Sunflower oil 1 tablespoon

Mix all ingredients in a small bottle. If possible have someone rub on your back, chest, legs, and neck.

Especially good when suffering from jet lag.

Lets Get Back To Sleep Massage Lotion

Marjoram 25 drops
Amyris 25 drops
Mandarin 25 drops
Massage Lotion 2 ounces

Blend the above essential oils in a glass bottle. Then add the essential oils to the 2 ounces of unscented massage lotion. Blend well, then massage your shoulders, neck and back.

Helpful Tip:

If a child or you have a problem falling asleep after a bad dream you can try using a little Frankincense, Melissa, or Roman Chamomile along with the old standby Lavender.

Just apply a few drops to the pillows on either end and the flip the pillow upside down.

As you drift off to sleep the essential oils should help you to relax and calm down for a better rest of the night sleep.

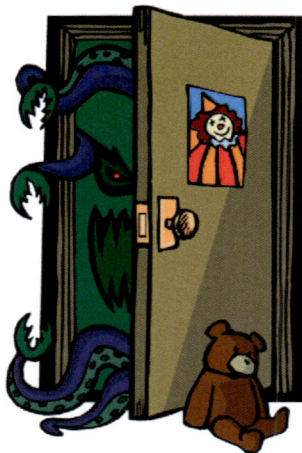

Shoo The Monsters Away Bedtime Spray

Roman Chamomile 12 drops
Lavender 12 drops
Orange 8 drops
Emulsifier 30 drops
Distilled water 8 ounces

Mix and spray on the pillow and in the air in the room. This mixture is good where "monsters" hide too!

Sleepy Time Bedtime Spray

Roman Chamomile 4 drops
Lavender 5 drops
Orange 4 drops

Blend with 4 ounces of distilled water or a linen spray in a spray bottle. Shake well before each use.

You can spray this on bed linens earlier in the day or you can spray in the room shortly before retiring.

If you have overnight guests, this may help them drift off to sleep more easily in your home.

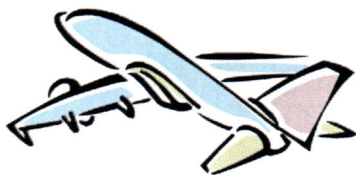

For Jet Lag –To Help You Drift Off To Sleep
Petitgrain 5 drops
Rose 5 drops
Myrtle 3 drops
Vanilla 2 drops
Sweet Almond 1 tablespoon

Blend together and either massage into the chest, back of neck, and shoulders.

You can also add this blend to a tub of warm water and enjoy.

If using this blend in the bath, please be careful as the Almond oil can make the tub slippery.

Simple Sleep Blend
Lavender 1 drop
Bergamot 1 drop

Place these on a tissue and place between your pillow case and pillow. Nighty night!!

Sweet Dreams—A Pillow Spray
Lavender 2 drops
Roman Chamomile 1 drop
Orange 1 drop
Ylang-Ylang 1 drop
Distilled Water 15 mls

Shake well and spray on pillow cases. Let dry. This is a great blend for out-of-town guests.

Sweet Slumber Sleepy Time
Sandalwood 6 drops
Neroli 2 drops
Ylang -Ylang 2 drops
Vetiver 1 drop
Coriander 1 drop
Jojoba 1 tablespoon

Blend these oils together and apply to your pulse points prior to bedtime.

Sleepy Time
Neroli 4 drops
Mandarin 3 drops
Oregano 3 drops
Lavender 3 drops
Carrier oil 1 tablespoon

Blend essential oils in carrier oil. Shake well and massage your legs, arms, and back (if you can find someone to do this for you!)

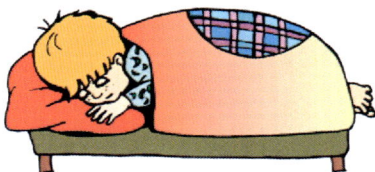

For Your "Snoring" Companion
Rosewood 4 drops
Geranium 4 drops
Basil 3 drops
Allspice 3 drops
Anise 3 drops
Lemongrass 3 drops
Carrier Oil 20 mls

Massage into upper chest, back of neck, across shoulders, and mid back.

Athlete's Foot Bath
Tea Tree 5 drops
Patchouli 4 drops
Myrrh 2 drops

Soak your feet in a small tub, where you have added the above oils. Let your feet soak for about 15 minutes. Dry your feet well.

Foot Deodorizing Powder
Sage 2 drops
Coriander 2 drops
Spearmint 2 drops
Talc Powder 2 ounces
Baking soda 1 tablespoon

Open the bottle of Talc Powder and add the baking soda. Shake well.

Then add the drops of essential oils to a cotton ball and drop inside the talc/baking soda bottle.

Shake well and let sit for a couple days before using. Apply to your feet and inside your shoes.

Athlete's Foot Powder
Lavender 15 drops
Peppermint 5 drops
Talc Powder 1 ounce

Add drops to a cotton pad and drop into the talc powder bottle. Shake well, several times over the next 24 hours.

The powder will be ready to use. Sprinkle on feet and between toes after bathing.

Dry between the toes well before applying powder.

Simple Foot Powder
Rosemary 5 drops
Tagetes 2 drops
Thyme 2 drops
Talc 5 ounces (by weight)

Shake well, let sit for 24 hours, shake again then use daily on your feet.

Dust on feet after showering, don't forget to spread your toes.

Just So You Know!

Fungal Infections– which is what Athletes foot is, can take several weeks to be controlled.

Using any essential oils blends consistently for several weeks to eliminate the fungal infection.

Alternate Blend For Fungus
Palmarosa 20 drops
Eucalyptus globulus 20 drops
Thyme 20 drops
Tea Tree 20 drops
Carrier oil 4 ounce

Blend well and apply 2-4 times a day for 10-14 days.

Discontinue after that if no improvement.

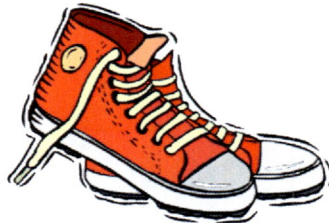

Stinky Sneaker Blend

Rosemary 25 drops
Lavender 20 drops
Tea Tree 20 drops
Baking soda 1/4 cup

Apply these essential oils to a cotton ball placed in a powder sifter bottle. Then add the 1/4 cup baking soda. Shake well and let blend for 24 hours.

After that, simply shake about 1 teaspoonful in each sneaker at the end of wearing them for the day. Leave over night, then shake out in the morning before putting them on again.

Freshen Up Those Sneakers

Lavender 40 drops
Tea Tree 40 drops
Baking soda 1/2 cup

Place in a glass jar and cover tightly. Stir or shake well to distribute the essential oils in with the baking soda.

Keep the jar sealed. Sprinkle in your smelly sneakers at night. Remember to empty your sneakers out in the morning before wearing

Soothing Sun Burn Bath

Lavender 8 drops
Roman Chamomile 2 drops
Helichrysum 2 drops
Peppermint 1 drop

Place the oils in the tub of cool water. Soak for 15-20 minutes.

Do not rub the burned areas. You can repeat this bath every few hours as necessary.

Sunburn Relief #1

Roman Chamomile 6 drops
Lavender 6 drops
Peppermint 3 drops
Sorbolene Cream 1 oz

Mix the above well, then add to the Sorbolene Cream
Blend well, then add:
Distilled water 1-2 teaspoons, to thin this blend down a little.

Apply to sunburned area as often as needed.

Sunburn Relief #2

Lavender 40 drops
Helichrysum 15 drops
Peppermint 1 drop
Jojoba 2 ounces

Blend well and use as needed on your sunburned skin.

Sunburn Relief #3

Lavender 60 drops
Helichrysum 25 drops
Jojoba 2 ounces
Aloe Vera Liquid 2 ounces

Blend and shake well and use as needed on your sunburned skin.

Add a few ice cubes to the water if you want to keep the water cool.

Use a small cup to gently poor water over hard to soak areas.

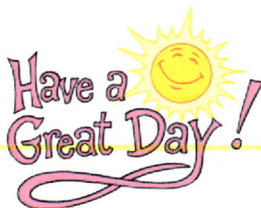

Have a Great Day!

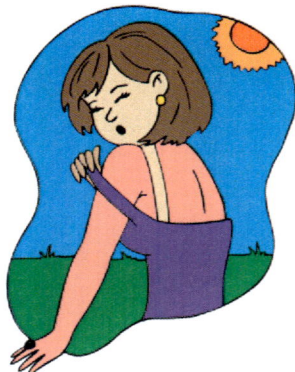

Sunburn Spray
Lavender 5 ml
Emulsifier 5 ml
Aloe Vera liquid 2 ounces

Blend essential oils and emulsifier in a PET spray topped bottle, then add the Aloe Vera.

Shake well and spray on sun-burned area.

Repeat as needed and STAY OUT OF THE SUN for the next few days!! You don't need to try to get a tan all in one day.

This is a spray that you may want to make up and keep in the refrigerator.

It can be used on any kind of burn that doesn't have broken skin. It is cool and will help the area to heal more quickly.

Sunburn Comfort
Lavender 10-15 drops
German Chamomile 2 drops
Jojoba oil.1 ounce

Blend well in a PET bottle and apply to the skin as needed.

After Sun Oil
Lavender 15 drops
Helichrysum 5 drops
Bergamot FCF 1 drop
Rose Otto 1 drop
Sesame oil 1 ounce
Jojoba 1 ounce

Blend all in a PET bottle then apply to the skin as desired.

Best if applied after a shower or bath. It will help sooth any minor sunburn and help to heal any damage done during the day.

Minty Lips
A very simple and easy chapped lip relief is to simply use a little Jojoba on your lips. It absorbs quickly and keeps then keeps them nice and soft. To 10 mls of Jojoba add 1 drop of Peppermint or Spearmint.

This mixture may give your lips a little tingle and warm feeling if this is too strong dilute with more Jojoba.

Try not to lick your lips for the first 10 or so minutes after you have applied this so the Jojoba can soak into the your lips.

Lip Soother
Lavender 3 drops
Roman Chamomile 2 drops
Macadamia Oil 10 mls
Roll-on Perfume Bottle

Blend the essential oils with the Macadamia oil and pour into a roll-on perfume bottle.
Apply to your lips as needed.

Brittle Nail Care

Lavender 2 drops
Sandalwood 2 drops
Cypress 2 drops
Almond Oil 1 ounce

Warm Almond oil in a small bowl, add the essential oils and submerge fingertips in the mixture for 10 minutes. You can do this 3-4 times a week to help soften them up.

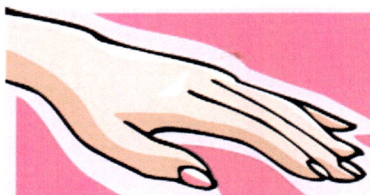

An Eczema Calming Bath

Chamomile 3 drops
Geranium 3 drops
Lemon 3 drops
Elemi 2 drops
Sandalwood 2 drops

Disperse all essential oils in the tub filled with warm water. Use this blend when your eczema flares up.

Sea Salt Anti-Fungal Bath

Lavender 4 drops
Tea tree 3 drops
Geranium 1 drop

Fill your bath tub, then add the essential oils. Add 1-2 cups of sea salts, mix well. Soak for a minimum of 20 minutes.

Be sure to dry your skin well, especially between your toes and other skin folds or cracks.

Corns and Calluses Softener

Tagetes 20 drops
Roman Chamomile 10 drops
Carrot seed 5 drops
Sunflower oil 2 tablespoons

Mix in a bottle and apply several drops to the corn twice daily.

Remember to soak your feet and vigorously rub the corn and calluses after soaking to help remove any of the dead skin.

You may need to use a pumice stone to help remove some of the dead, thickened skin.

Continue to use the above blend, periodically, once you have the corn and/or calluses gone to help prevent them from returning.

Compress For Varicose Veins

Cypress 8 drops
Lemon 5 drops
Bergamot 5 drops
Cool Water

Mix oil into cool water, wring out a cotton cloth in mixture and place over area. Leave compress on for 15 minutes, then replace. Do this 2-3 times daily.

Arthritic Joint Soaking Bath

Juniper berry 4 drops
Lavender 2 drops
Cypress 2 drops
Rosemary 2 drops

Add this blend to a bath while filling or just after filling the tub and soak for 20-30 minutes.

Reducing Cellulite Massage

Pine 12 drops
Juniper Berry 12 drops
Fennel 12 drops
Lime 12 drops
Thyme 12 drops
Sunflower Oil 2 ounces

Blend all the essential oils together and add to the sunflower oil. Shake well.

Then massage this formula into the cellulite areas, work deeply into the tissue to help smooth bumpy and dimpled skin.

After Bath Anti-Cellulite Massage Oil

Follow your bath with a few drops of this alternative body oil to the affected areas.

Lemon 15 drops
Cypress 15 drops
Carrotseed 5 drops
Juniper 5 drops
Jojoba 1/4 teaspoon
Sweet Almond 1 ounce

Apply this to the areas affected.
Then use a dry brush to increase circulation.

This will aid in the elimination of toxins. Remember to drink plenty of fresh water.

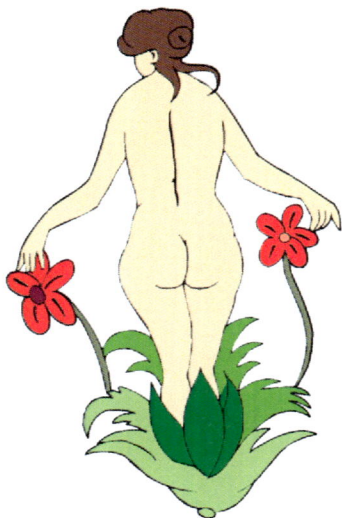

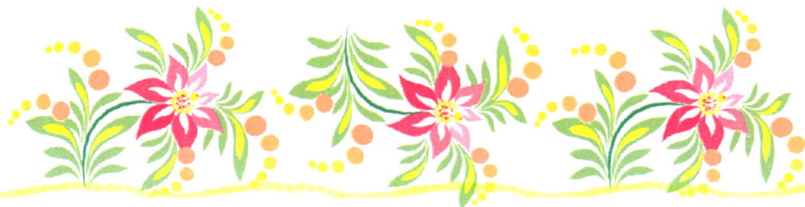

Cellulite Massage

Eucalyptus 40 drops
Lemon 40 drops
Cedarwood 40 drops
Sage 40 drops
Cypress 40 drops
Niaouli 40 drops
Hazelnut oil 3 1/2 ounces

Blend well in a PET bottle. Massage into affected areas 2-3 times a day for up to 30 days.

Due to the citrus oils in this blend, avoid direct sunlight for at least 2 hours after applying.

Citrus oils can cause some people to have a photo sensitization reaction with their skin.

PART THREE
The Index

LIST OF RECIPES

List By Category

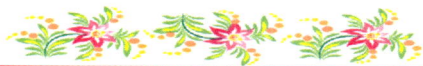

NOTES

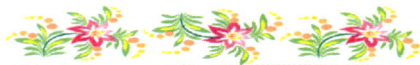

NOTES

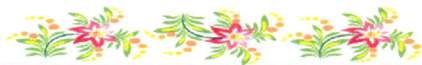

NOTES

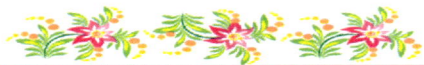

NOTES